Radiology for Anaesthetists

Conrad Wittram MB ChB, DMRD, FRCR
*Lecturer, Department of Radiodiagnosis, University of Liverpool
and Honorary Senior Registrar, The Royal Liverpool University
Hospital NHS Trust, UK*

Graham Whitehouse FRCP, FRCR, DMRD, AKC
*Professor of Diagnostic Radiology, Head of the Department of Radiodiagnosis,
University of Liverpool and Honorary Consultant Radiologist,
The Royal Liverpool University Hospital NHS Trust, UK*

ARNOLD

A member of the Hodder Headline Group
LONDON • SYDNEY • AUCKLAND
Co-published in the USA by
Oxford University Press, Inc., New York

© 1996 Conrad Wittram and Graham Whitehouse

First published in Great Britain in 1996 by
Arnold, a member of the Hodder Headline Group,
338 Euston Road, London NW1 3BH

Co-published in the United States of America by
Oxford University Press Inc.,
198 Madison Avenue, New York, NY 10016
Oxford is a registered trademark of Oxford University Press

Whilst the advice and information in this book is believed to be true and
accurate at the date of going to press, neither the authors nor the publisher
can accept any legal responsibility or liability for any errors or omissions
that may be made.

British Library Cataloguing in Publication Data
A catalogue record for this book is available from the British Library

Library of Congress Cataloging-in-Publication Data
A catalog record for this book is available from the Library of Congress

ISBN 0 340 55790 7

1 2 3 4 5   96 97 98 99

Typeset in 10/12 pt Palatino by GreenGate Publishing Services, Tonbridge, Kent
Printed and bound in Great Britain by the Bath Press, Avon

Contents

Preface

Anaesthetists, as well as other medical practitioners involved in critical care, will hopefully find this book to be a useful guide when interpreting radiographs and determining the appropriate use of diagnostic imaging in their practice. *Radiology for Anaesthetists* is also aimed at helping trainee radiologists to prepare for specialist examinations.

The introductory chapter includes information on radiographic technique and anatomy, together with a systematic approach to the interpretation of chest radiographs. A brief overview of other imaging techniques is also presented. The second part of the book consists of 80 questions and answers, following a similar format to the objective structured clinical examination component of the Fellowship examination of the Royal College of Anaesthetists. The answers include a description of radiological findings, management principles and, where relevant, discussion or a differential diagnosis. The cases chosen for this interactive approach cover many of the conditions that anaesthetists are likely to come across in their day-to-day practice.

We hope that this book will prove to be interesting and challenging as well as educational, and that it will ultimately benefit patient care.

Conrad Wittram
Graham Whitehouse
1995

Acknowledgements

We acknowledge the patience and encouragement of our wives Kate and Jackie. We wish to express our gratitude to our many colleagues in Liverpool who contributed to the selection of cases. Special thanks are due to Mrs Joan Scott for producing the manuscript and Mr David Adkins for the preparation of the illustrations.

Erratum: Arnold wishes to apologise to the reader for an error regarding the index. From page 28 onwards, all index page references should read two pages forward from the page given. This is due to the late insertion of a part title.

1 Chest Radiology

Chest radiographs account for a third of all radiological examinations. Indications for chest radiography are given in Appendix A.

The posteroanterior (PA) chest radiograph

Technique

The patient stands erect with his anterior chest wall against the vertical film holder. The X-ray tube is situated 2m behind the patient. The chin is elevated, while the shoulders are rotated forwards in order to prevent the scapulae from overlapping the lung fields. The exposure is made during full inspiration. The X-ray beam is aimed at the fourth thoracic vertebra. A voltage of 70 kVp will give good bony detail and will demonstrate calcification. Improved visibility of detail within the mediastinum and lungs is obtained by using a higher voltage, such as 125–150 kVp. However, bones and calcification are not so clearly seen with the higher voltage. In heavier subjects, greater detail is obtained by using a grid to minimize scattered radiation.

Assessing the quality of a PA chest radiograph

1. *Markings:* Ensure that the patient's name and the date of examination are correct. Check that a right or left side marker is present.
2. *Centring:* The medial ends of the clavicles should be equidistant from the spinous processes in the midline of the upper thoracic spine. The lungs should normally have an equal degree of translucency to each other. Rotation of the patient causes the lungs to have a difference in translucency which may mimic pulmonary disease. A normal hilum may appear unduly prominent when there is rotation of the patient. Rotation to the left may cause apparent displacement and enlargement of the heart.
3. *Inspiration:* If the radiograph is taken at full inspiration in a normal subject, the mid-point of the right hemidiaphragm should lie between the anterior ends of the fifth and seventh ribs. An inadequate inspiratory effort gives a false appearance of cardiac enlargement and abnormal shadowing in the lung bases. Obesity, a distended abdomen or postoperative pain may cause limited inspiration.
4. *Penetration:* Faint visualization of the thoracic spine and intervertebral discs ensures that the pulmonary vessels behind the heart are well seen.

Analysis of the PA chest radiograph *(Figures 1, 2 and 3)*

The chest radiograph should be scanned in a systematic manner. It does not matter where you start or the order in which you assess the features, as long as you have a thorough and consistent approach. The following scheme begins by assessing the radiographic quality and looking at the corners of the film. After an initial quick review of the lungs, they are carefully assessed region by region. The diaphragms and pleura, then the upper abdomen are next assessed. The heart and mediastinum are then reviewed from below upwards.

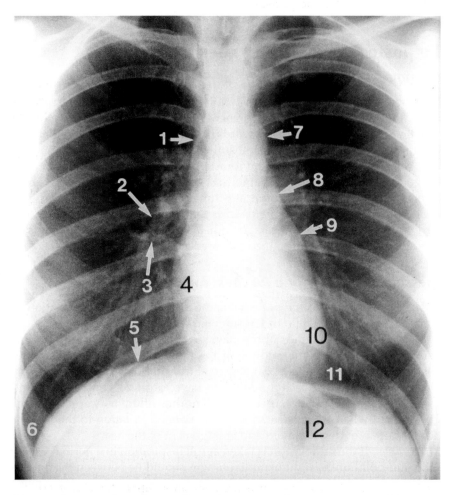

Figure 1 The normal PA chest radiograph. 1 = superior vena cava; 2 = right pulmonary artery; 3 = right upper lobe pulmonary vein; 4 = right atrium; 5 = right hemidiaphragm; 6 = right lateral costophrenic angle; 7 = aortic arch; 8 = pulmonary trunk; 9 = auricular appendage of left atrium; 10 = left ventricle; 11 = left cardiophrenic angle; 12 = gas in gastric fundus.

The bones are checked and finally the soft tissues of the chest wall.

Radiographic quality:
The assessment of radiographic quality in regard to penetration, rotation and inspiration have been described above.

Additional information:
Check the side markers. Look at the name of the patient and the date the radiograph was taken. Sometimes the time of day will also be given. The patient's age will often be included on the radiograph. See if there are any other radiographs for comparison.

Lungs

The lungs are conveniently divided into three zones:

1. Upper zone – apex down to lower border of anterior end of second rib.
2. Mid-zone – between lower borders of anterior ends of second and fourth ribs.
3. Lower zone – between lower border of anterior end of fourth rib down to diaphragm.

Compare corresponding zones in each lung. The distribution of blood vessels should be equal between the two zones at each of the three levels. The lungs should be equally translucent. Normally, the only structures seen within the lungs are the blood vessels and fissures. Any other opacities are likely to be

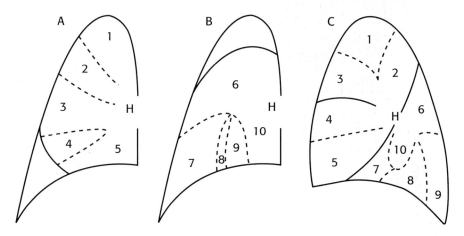

Figure 2 Illustrations of the position of the right lung segments seen on the AP (A,B) and lateral (C) chest radiographs. A shows the segments in the upper and middle lobes only. B shows the segments in the lower lobes. C shows all the segments in the lateral projection. H = hila; 1 = apical segment of the right upper lobe (RUL); 2 = posterior segment of RUL; 3 = anterior segment of RUL; 4 = lateral segment of RML; 5 = medial segment of RML; 6 = apical segment of RLL; 7 = anterior basal segment of RLL; 8 = lateral basal segment of RLL; 9 = posterior basal segment of RLL; 10 = medial basal segment of RLL.

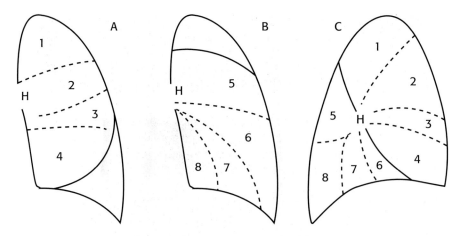

Figure 3 Illustrations of the position of the left lung segments on the AP (A,B) and lateral (C) chest radiographs. A shows the segments in the upper lobe and lingula only. B shows the segments in the lower lobes only. C shows all the segments in the lateral projection. H = hila; 1 = apicoposterior segment of left upper lobe (LUL); 2 = anterior segment of LUL; 3 = superior segment of lingula; 4 = inferior segment of lingula; 5 = apical segment of LLL; 6 = anterior basal segment of LLL; 7 = lateral basal segment of LLL; 8 = posterior basal segment of LLL.

pathological in nature. The walls of the peripheral bronchi are not usually visible. Apart from pleural and pulmonary disease, a relative decrease in radiolucency of one lung compared to the other may also be caused by rotation or difference in chest wall soft tissues.

While observing the mid-zones, it is convenient to asses the *hila*. The normal hilar opacities are produced entirely by blood vessels and should be of similar radiodensity. Hilar lymph nodes are not visible unless they are pathologically enlarged. The normal hila typically form the shape of a letter V lying on its side, the upper limb being the upper lobe veins crossing the hilum to reach the left atrium. The lower limb is the lower lobe branch of the pulmonary artery. The mid-point of the hilum lies at the apex of the V, at the level of the horizontal fissure and the sixth rib in the mid-axillary line. The mid-point of the left hilum lies 1–1.5 cm higher than that of the right hilum.

Diaphragms

The diaphragms are convex, the curve being assessed by measuring the distance between the highest point of the hemidiaphragm and a line joining the costophrenic and cardiophrenic angles. This measurement is normally at least 1.5 cm. The right hemidiaphragm is usually 1.5–2 cm higher than the left. A difference of more than 3 cm may be significant. However, the hemidiaphragms may normally lie at the same level, although this typically occurs with hyperinflation. The left hemidiaphragm may be higher than the right, particularly when the stomach or splenic flexure is distended by gas.

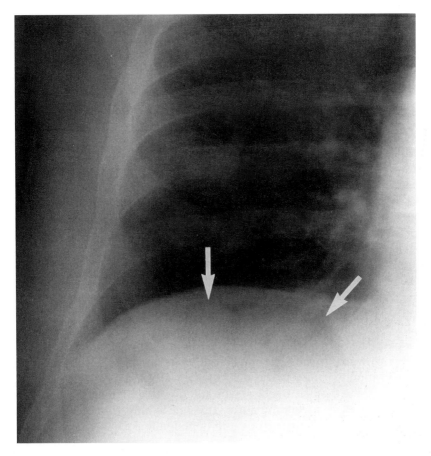

Figure 4 Chilaiditi's syndrome. The subphrenic region in an asymptomatic patient shows faint airfilled loops of colon interposed between the liver and right hemidiaphragm (arrows). Note haustrations on the colonic segment.

Upper abdomen

In the appropriate clinical context, check for pneumoperitoneum. Air may remain in the peritoneal cavity for up to three weeks after abdominal (and occasionally thoracic) surgery. As a normal variant, bowel may be interposed between the liver and right hemidiaphragm (Chilaiditi's syndrome) (Figure 4).

Heart and mediastinum

From above downwards, the right mediastinal border consists of innominate vessels, superior vena cava, right atrium and sometimes a small part of the IVC. In older patients, a prominent ascending aorta may form part of the right border. The left mediastinal border, from above downwards, consists of the subclavian artery, the aortic knuckle, the pulmonary trunk, which may be particularly prominent in young women, the left atrial appendage and the left ventricle. The azygos vein lies in the angle between the right main bronchus and trachea. It is most prominent on supine radiographs. On erect radiographs the azygos vein is less than 10 mm and decreases in size with inspiration.

The mediastinal and cardiac borders are normally sharply defined, except where the inferior cardiac border abuts onto the left hemidiaphragm. The epicardiac fat pads occupy the cardiophrenic angles and, when prominent, may simulate cardiac enlargement. Usually two-thirds of the heart lie to the left of the midline and one-third to the right. The maximum cardiac diameter on a PA chest radiograph is usually less than 13.5 cm, more than 15.5 cm indicating cardiomegaly. The maximum difference in transverse cardiac diameter between diastole and systole is not more than 1.5 cm. An increase of more than 1.5 cm on serial radiographs is therefore abnormal. Heart size can also be expressed as the cardiothoracic ratio, i.e. the ratio between the maximum transverse diameter of the heart and the internal thoracic diameter at the level of the costophrenic angles. In a normal adult, on full inspiration, the cardiothoracic ratio should be no more than 0.5.

The trachea is a vertical translucent band, seen from the larynx down to the carina. While its upper part lies in the midline, the lower portion is deviated slightly to the right by the aortic arch. The trachea should be of constant calibre and 1.5–2 cm wide throughout its length, although it becomes less distinct in its lower part. The right tracheal margin, known as the right paratracheal stripe, is traced downwards to the right main bronchus in 60% of adults and is normally less than 5 mm in diameter. The left paratracheal stripe is rarely seen.

Overlying the thoracic trachea is the anterior junction line, where the lungs meet anterior to the ascending aorta. This line is only 1mm thick and curves slightly from right to left. The posterior junction line is where the lungs meet behind the oesophagus and is straight or convexly curved to the left. It is 2mm wide and runs from the lung apices to the aortic knuckle. These junctional lines are seen only occasionally.

Paraspinal lines, usually 1–2 mm wide, run adjacent to the vertebral bodies and are the posterior parts of the medial pleura seen end on.

Thoracic cage

The ribs are examined throughout their length, one at a time from above downwards. The shoulder girdles are usually visible on a PA chest radiograph.

Soft tissues of chest wall

Nipple shadows are sometimes seen, in males as well as females, as rounded nodules overlying the lower zones and 0.5–1.5 cm in size. Both nipple are usually visible and often appear least well defined in their superomedial aspects. If doubt persists, the radiograph should be repeated with radio-opaque nipple markers. A mastectomy is usually obvious on a chest radiograph and may cause increased translucency of the ipsilateral lung. Asymmetry of pectoralis muscles may cause similar appearances.

Review areas

Finally, it is recommended that a further check is made of areas where pathology may be easily missed:

1. *Lung apices*: Pneumothorax, subtle TB and small Pancoast tumours may be obscured by the upper ribs.
2. *Hila*: Subtle changes in position, density, size and contour of the hila may be the manifestation of important lesions such as bronchial carcinoma.
3. *Behind the heart:* Metastases, left lower lobe collapse and hiatus hernia are examples of lesions which occur within the cardiac outline.

The chest radiograph in the elderly

With increasing age, there is shrinkage of the transverse thoracic diameter. This will cause an increase in the cardiothoracic ratio. At the same time, there will be an increase in the anteroposterior thoracic diameter with the development of a kyphosis. Fibrosis and calcification from old TB, pleural thickening and linear scars may be residual evidence of previous infections.

The aortic arch becomes dilated and elongated, resulting in prominence of the aortic knuckle. Calcification of the aortic arch is common and there may be calcification within the aortic and, less frequently, the mitral valve. Unfolding of the innominate and subclavian arteries causes widening of the superior mediastinum, but without tracheal narrowing. Calcification may also occur in cartilaginous rings of the trachea and main bronchi, almost exclusively in elderly women.

Osteopenia may cause fracture of vertebral bodies and ribs. Costal cartilage calcification becomes prominent in old age.

The lateral chest radiograph (Figure 5)

When screening patients for chest disease, it is common practice to obtain only a PA radiograph and not to routinely include a lateral radiograph. However, some pleural and pulmonary lesions may only be visible on the lateral radiograph, particularly when they lie behind the heart or are hidden in the costophrenic recess on the PA radiograph. In general, the lateral chest radiograph is used to evaluate the site, size, morphology and nature of abnormalities seen on the PA radiograph. The lateral projection chosen is that which brings the abnormality closer to the film. If there is no obvious abnormality on the PA radiograph, a left lateral projection is obtained because more of the left lung than the right lung is obscured on the PA projection. A lateral radiograph gives no problem in a fit patient, the arms being elevated to a vertical position. An ill patient may only be able to raise his arms to a right angle, clasping the hands behind the head with the elbows parallel.

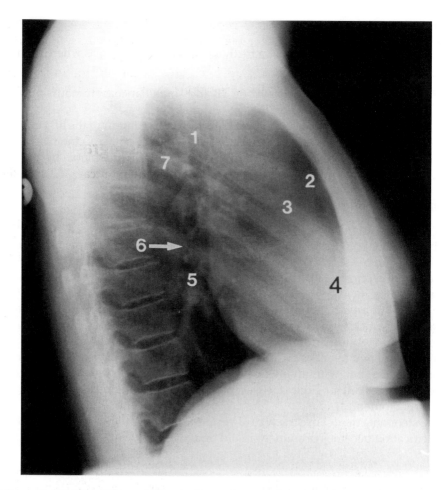

Figure 5 The normal lateral chest radiograph. 1 = air in the trachea; 2 = transradiency of apposition of lungs anterior to the heart; 3 = pulmonary outflow tract; 4 = region of right ventricle; 5 = lower lobe artery; 6 = lower lobe bronchus; 7 = aortic arch.

Radiological anatomy

Both diaphragms are normally visible. The left hemidiaphragm can be distinguished from the right by the gastric air bubble which lies immediately underneath it. In addition, the anterior part of the left hemidiaphragm is obscured where it is in contact with the inferior surface of the heart.

The anterior border of the heart comprises the right ventricle, above which lies the ascending part of the aortic arch. The translucency between the sternum and ascending aorta is where there is apposition of the right and left lungs. The trachea is seen as a translucent band running downwards from the thoracic inlet and crossed in the upper chest by the transverse part of the aortic arch. The lower end of the trachea is overlaid by the pulmonary artery. The hila tend to be superimposed on a lateral radiograph. The descending part of the aortic arch is also visible. The horizontal fissure is seen as a fine line running forwards from the hilar density. Parts of the oblique fissures are usually visible. Normally, the thoracic vertebrae appear to become progressively less dense from top to bottom.

The portable anteroposterior (AP) radiograph

The portable chest radiograph, taken at the bedside or occasionally in the operating theatre, is inevitably of inferior quality to the formal PA radiograph. The radiographic film, in its lightproof cassette, lies immediately under the supine patient or behind the sitting patient. The divergence of the X-ray beam inevitably results in magnification of anteriorly situated structures in the chest. Increasing the distance between the X-ray tube and the patient to 1 m or

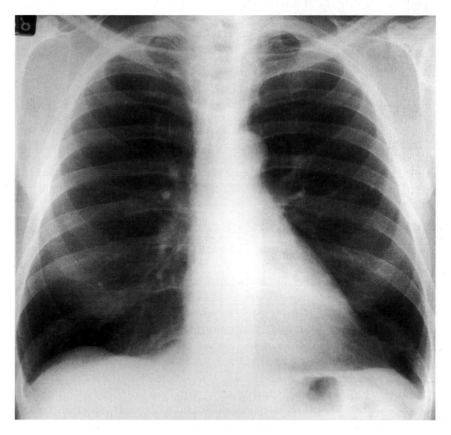

Figure 6 The normal erect PA chest radiograph of a male patient demonstrates a cardiothoracic ratio of 0.40.

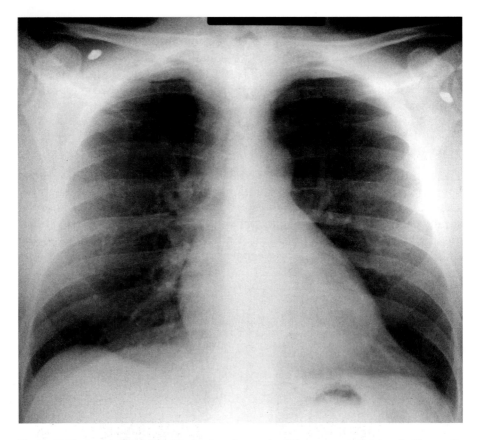

Figure 7 The normal supine AP chest radiograph of the same patient as in Figure 6 demonstrates a cardiothoracic ratio of 0.46 and upper lobe venous dilatation, mimicking pulmonary venous hypertension.

more reduces the degree of divergence. Nevertheless, the heart and superior mediastinum are magnified by approximately 15–20% on an AP radiograph, compared with 5% in the conventional PA chest radiograph. The clavicles and arterial ends of the ribs, being furthest from the film, are magnified and less well defined than the posterior parts of the ribs.

There is inevitably a reduced inspiratory excursion in a patient who is lying down or semirecumbent in bed, compounding the cardiac magnification and causing difficulties in evaluating the underinflated lung bases. In the supine position, upward rotation of the liver may cause elevation of the right hemidiaphragm.

Pulmonary blood volume is increased by 30% in recumbency, compared to the erect position. The pulmonary vessels therefore appear larger on a supine chest radiograph. This is especially so in the upper lobes where vascular dilatation is enhanced by removal of the effect of gravity, mimicking pulmonary venous hypertension (Figures 6 and 7).

A sick patient, propped up in bed or lying supine, is more likely to be rotated than a fit and co-operative standing subject, further increasing artefactural difficulties. Pleural effusions may diffuse through the pleural space and become inconspicuous, while pneumothoraces may not be visible on a supine radiograph.

Supplementary radiographic projections

Lordotic projection

An angled view of the upper part of the chest is used to show the lung apices and superior mediastinum to better effect, the clavicles and uppermost ribs being projected in an upward direction (Figures 8 and 9). A lordotic projection may occasionally be used to demonstrate a right middle lobe collapse. As originally described, the lordotic view is taken in the AP direction. The patient leans backwards with the interscapular region touching the film holder. A

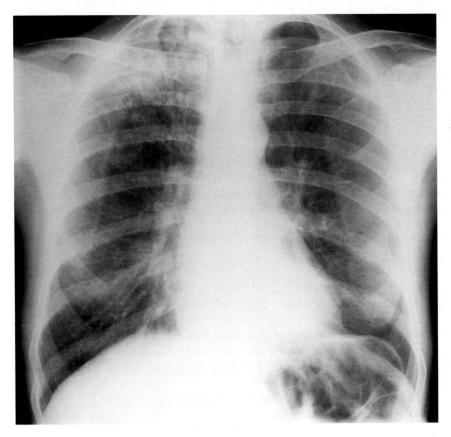

Figure 8 The AP chest radiograph of a patient with tuberculous consolidation in the right apex.

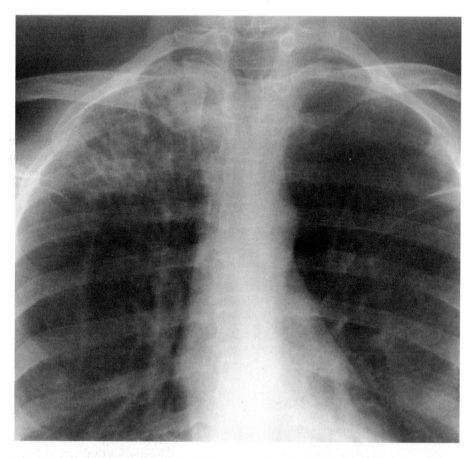

Figure 9 The lordotic radiograph of the same patient projects the clavicle upwards, revealing more detail of the apical segment. Cavitation can now be excluded with confidence.

more convenient method is an AP projection with the X-ray tube angled 15° towards the head and the patient erect.

AP projection

An erect AP projection is sometimes helpful in determining whether or not an opacity at the same level as a rib actually lies within the rib or in the underlying lung.

Inspiration and expiration radiographs

Radiographs taken in full inspiration and expiration are used:

1. *to demonstrate air trapping:* When air trapping is widespread, as in asthma and emphysema, there is very slight diaphragmatic movement and limited

density changes in the lungs at the extremes of respiration. With local air trapping, for instance from bronchial obstruction or lobar emphysema, the expiration radiograph will show limited ipsilateral diaphragmatic elevation, mediastinal shift towards the contralateral hemithorax and relative absence of density changes in the obstructed part of the lung.

2. *in suspected pneumothorax:* When the visceral pleura is not visible on the inspiration radiograph or the appearances are equivocal, the pneumothorax should be more clearly seen on an expiration radiograph. This is because the volume of the pneumothorax is relatively greater than the lung volume on expiration, resulting in a wider gap between visceral and parietal pleura.

In an obvious pneumothorax, a substantial decrease in the lung volume on expiration indicates that the defect in the visceral pleura is closed or small, whereas only slight change in lung volume indicates an open pleural defect.

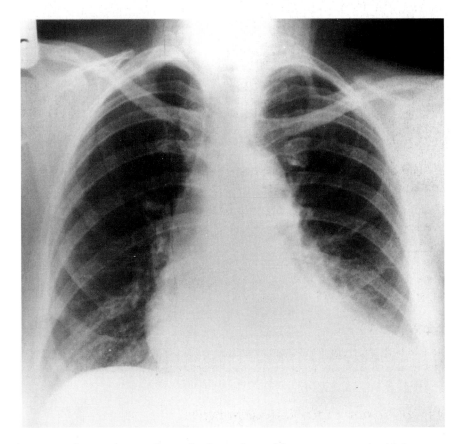

Figure 10 The AP chest radiograph of a patient with an apparent raised left hemidiaphragm. The apex of the diaphragm is more lateral than normal, suggesting a subpulmonary effusion.

Lateral decubitus radiograph

The patient lies on one side with the film cassette against their back and a horizontal beam impinging upon their anterior chest wall. Lateral decubitus radiographs are useful in showing:

1. *small pleural effusions;* less than 100ml of pleural fluid may be visible in this projection, whereas an erect radiograph seldom shows effusions of less than 300 ml.
2. *subpulmonary pleural effusions,* which may be difficult to distinguish from an elevated hemidiaphragm on an erect radiograph, run freely in the pleural space when the ipsilateral side is dependent (Figures 10 and 11).
3. *positional changes* of an air–fluid level or a loose body, for instance within a cavity.

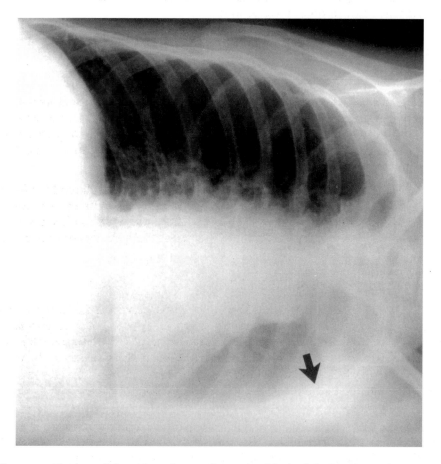

Figure 11 The lateral decubitus chest radiograph with the left side dependent shows the pleural fluid has run freely within the pleural space (arrow), confirming the diagnosis of a pleural effusion.

Oblique radiographs

These are useful in showing pleural plaques in asbestos exposure, although the optimal degree of obliquity is best chosen during fluoroscopy.

Linear tomography

This is a radiographic technique in which detail is shown in sectional planes of the body. Structural detail on either side of the chosen plane is minimized or removed. Tomography has to a large extent been replaced by computed tomography (CT). If CT is not available, linear tomography may be used:

1. to provide further detail on pulmonary nodules and masses than is seen on standard radiographs.
2. in hilar enlargement to distinguish between vascular prominence and lymphadenopathy or other mass lesions.

The paediatric chest

Technique

In the *neonate*, satisfactory radiographs may be obtained in incubators with a film cassette under the patient. An experienced radiographer will be able to judge the exposure at the point of maximum inspiration. In an adequate inspiration, the right hemidiaphragm will be at the level of the posterior part of the right eighth rib.

Below the age of five, an assistant, preferably the mother, holds the child in front of a film cassette within a chest stand. There is very little difference between AP and PA projections in a small child. A high kV technique is often used. *After the age of five*, it is usually possible to obtain a PA radiograph, as in the adult.

Radiographic anatomy in a child

Normally the *thymus* causes a widening of the superior mediastinum in infants and young children. The thymus may have a 'sail-like' configuration, particularly on the right side. The lateral margin is undulated, due to indentations from the ribs. The thymus may shrink in response to stress or steroid therapy. Ultrasound may be helpful in distinguishing cystic lesions from normal homogeneous thymic tissue when there is questionable thymic enlargement.

Heart size

In infants and small children, the cardiothoracic ratio can exceed 50% and cardiomegaly should be diagnosed with caution in this age group.

Trachea

Kinking of the trachea to the right is frequently seen when there has been a shallow inspiration.

Soft tissues

A prominent anterior axillary fold across the chest wall can mimic a pneumothorax. Skin folds can also cause confusing opacities.

Pleural effusions

In children, pleural effusions typically cause separation of the lung from the chest wall, with preservation of the costophrenic angles and accentuation of lung fissures.

Radiological procedures that may be helpful in evaluating the chest

Fluoroscopy

This is useful in assessing:

1. *diaphragmatic movement,* particularly in an elevated hemidiaphragm when phrenic nerve palsy is suspected. Sniffing, rather than normal respiration, is best for eliciting the paradoxical movement of the diaphragm which occurs in this condition.
2. *mediastinal movement,* especially in children with obstructive emphysema when the mediastinum swings to the non-obstructed side.
3. *localization* of pulmonary and pleural abnormalities seen on standard radiographs.

Barium swallow

Indications for a barium swallow include:

1. investigation of oesophageal causes of lung disease: particularly aspiration secondary to, for instance, pharyngeal palsy or pouch, hiatus hernia, achalasia and oesophageal obstruction.
2. investigation of chest pain: to demonstrate gastro-oesophageal reflux and oesophagitis.
3. supplementary to investigation of upper alimentary tract in haematemesis.
4. demonstration of tracheo-oesophageal fistula in neonates.

In cases of suspected oesophageal rupture, water-soluble contrast medium is initially used as extravasated barium may cause mediastinal granulomata.

Bronchography

For many years, bronchography was used to demonstrate bronchiectasis and to investigate patients with haemoptysis of obscure origin. Nowadays, bronchiography has been replaced by CT in evaluating the presence and extent of bronchiectasis. Fibreoptic bronchoscopy has replaced bronchography in the investigation of segmental and subsegmental lesions.

Angiography

Pulmonary arteriography

The main indications are the diagnosis of pulmonary embolism and occasionally the evaluation of congenital vascular abnormalities such as arteriovenous malformations and anomalous pulmonary venous drainage.

Arch aortography

This is the definitive diagnostic method in suspected traumatic damage to the aortic arch, although CT and especially MRI may provide sufficient information.

In aortic dissection, CT has a high exclusion value but MRI gives complete diagnostic information in a non-invasive manner. However, aortography may still be used when these methods are not available or to demonstrate subphrenic extension or a dissection.

Bronchial arteriography

Bronchial arteriography may be used to investigate the source of severe haemoptysis in bronchiectasis and may be combined with embolization.

Venography

Ascending venography, following the introduction of contrast medium via a vein on the dorsum of the foot, allows a full evaluation of the deep venous system of the lower limb, including iliac veins and inferior vena cava. Ultrasound, particularly colour flow Doppler, is an accurate method of evaluating the leg veins for diagnosing or excluding thrombosis. However, it permits only a limited assessment of the veins below the knee, although this limitation may not affect clinical management.

2 The Abnormal Chest Radiograph

When evaluating an abnormality on a chest radiograph, having applied the scheme described above, it is important (1) to define the location and extent of the lesion and (2) to describe the lesion using appropriate terminology. In regard to location, a lesion may arise from the chest wall, pleura, lung or mediastinum.

Chest wall lesions

Most chest wall lesions arise in ribs and a bony abnormality will usually be visible on radiography. Chest wall lesions may displace pleura; the margin of the lesion abutting the lung is rounded and sharply defined. Examples of chest wall lesions include rib metastases, soft tissue tumours, e.g. lipoma and fibroma, haematoma from surgery and other trauma.

Pleural lesions

Typically, pleural fluid on a PA radiograph obliterates the lateral costophrenic angle and, when large, a variable length of the hemidiaphragm. The upper margin of a pleural effusion is concave. A small effusion will collect in the most dependent portion of the pleural space, i.e. the posterior costophrenic angle, and will be visible on a lateral radiograph but may not be apparent in the PA projection.

Pleural effusions may extend into the fissures. When an effusion is loculated in a fissure it may appear as a rounded mass in the frontal projection, but its fissural site is usually readily apparent on a lateral radiograph.

Massive pleural effusions may cause complete opacification of a hemithorax and shift of the mediastinum to the contralateral side. Lack of displacement means that the ipsilateral lung is totally collapsed or the mediastinum is anchored by malignant infiltration.

A subpulmonary effusion will mimic an elevated diaphragm, although the apex of its convex upper surface is usually more lateral than it is on a hemidiaphragm. In a pneumothorax, the lung collapses towards the hilum, so that the visceral pleura is clearly visible, especially on an expiration film.

Pulmonary lesions

Increased density of the lung is situated in the air spaces or the interstitium, or both.

Air space disease

1. *Alveolar or acinar shadowing:* When an acinus is filled with fluid, it appears as a rounded nodular opacity, approximately 5mm in size. Confluence of these opacities results in larger areas of homogeneous shadowing with ill-defined margins, obscuring the pulmonary vessels.
2. *Air bronchogram:* When the bronchi remain patent and do not contain fluid, but are surrounded by consolidated lung, they appear as radiolucent branching structures. This is an air bronchogram (Figure 12). Causes of alveolar shadowing include pulmonary oedema, pneumonia, pulmonary

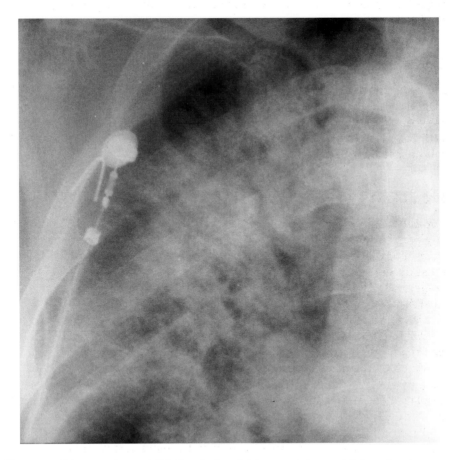

Figure 12 Pneumonic consolidation in the right upper lobe containing air bronchograms.

haemorrhage, infiltration, e.g. alveolar cell carcinoma, hyaline membrane disease and aspiration.

3. *Silhouette sign:* A silhouette is normally formed around the border of an anatomical structure, namely the heart, mediastinum or diaphragm, in sharp contrast to the adjacent airfilled lung. An airless intrathoracic lesion, such as a consolidated or collapsed portion of lung or adjacent pleural effusion, will efface the silhouette of the normal structures. This loss of silhouette is known as the *silhouette sign.* This important sign permits localization of lesions on the chest radiograph. As we have seen, a pleural effusion will obliterate the diaphragm and sometimes the mediastinal contour. However, the silhouette sign is particularly useful in localizing pulmonary consolidation. For instance, consolidation obscuring a hemidiaphragm will be in a lower lobe; if the right cardiac border is

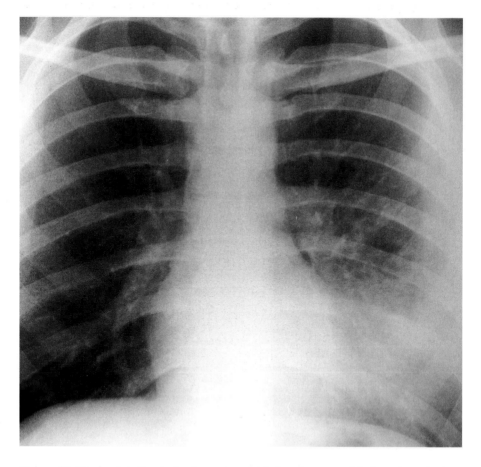

Figure 13 PA chest radiograph of a patient with lingular consolidation obscuring the normal left heart border, i.e. the silhouette sign.

obscured then it is the right middle lobe. Lingular consolidation obscures the left heart border (Figure 13) and left upper lobe consolidation will be indistinct from the aortic knuckle.

4. *Collapse (atelectasis):* The radiological signs of lobar collapse include:

   1. displacement of fissures,
   2. loss of aeration, which results in increased radiodensity and adjacent structures may become obscured (silhouette sign again);
   3. hilar displacement – upwards in upper lobe collapse and downwards in lower lobe collapse;
   4. compensatory hyperinflation: the uninvolved lobes may show increased translucency and their vessels become widely separated, due to hyperinflation.

Linear atelectasis or collapse, often seen in the lung bases of postoperative patients (Figure 14), is usually due to a combination of shallow inspiration and mucus plugs within the small bronchi. However, other pathological changes, including lung fibrosis and pleural reactions, may cause this appearance.

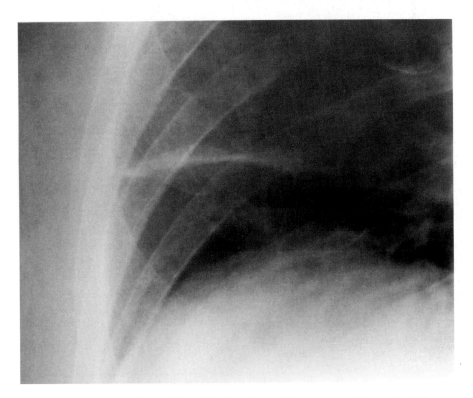

Figure 14 A close-up view of the right lung base of a postoperative patient demonstrates linear atelectasis.

Interstitial lung disease

Thickening of the interstitium produces a variety of linear, reticular and nodular shadowing. Interstitial pulmonary oedema is the commonest cause, fibrosing alveolitis typically involves the lower lobes but sarcoidosis and most pneumoconioses usually spare the bases. Infections which may cause interstitial lung disease include tuberculosis, viruses and pneumocystis.

Small nodular shadows less than 5mm in diameter are described as *miliary*. TB is a particularly important cause. Metastases, sarcoidosis and pneumoconiosis are other causes.

Larger nodular shadows are often due to metastases.

Linear shadowing

Interstitial lines are either A or B lines. B lines are horizontal, non-branching fine lines at the periphery of the lung, mostly in the lower zones. They are

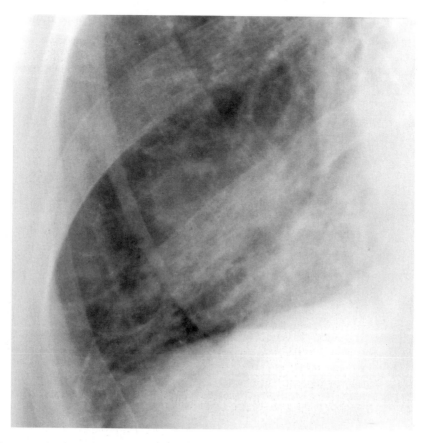

Figure 15 A close-up view of the right lung base of a patient with congestive cardiac failure shows septal (Kerley B) lines running to the edge of the lung.

usually due to fluid around distended lymphatics in interlobular septa (Figure 15). A lines are more centrally situated, usually around the hila, and are also due to oedema around lymphatics. Interstitial lines occur in cardiogenic and non-cardiogenic pulmonary oedema, lymphangitis carcinomatosis, pneumoconiosis and sarcoidosis.

Reticulonodular shadowing (honeycombing) is due to interstitial thickening around small air cysts. Apart from fibrosing alveolitis, this appearance occurs in many other diseases including sarcoidosis and pneumoconiosis (Figure 16).

Solitary pulmonary nodule

The majority of solitary pulmonary nodules are granulomas, primary lung tumours or metastases. Radiological appearances which favour benignity are a well-defined edge, calcification within the mass and no change in radiological appearance over two years. Malignant lesions tend to have an irregular margin and invade surrounding structures.

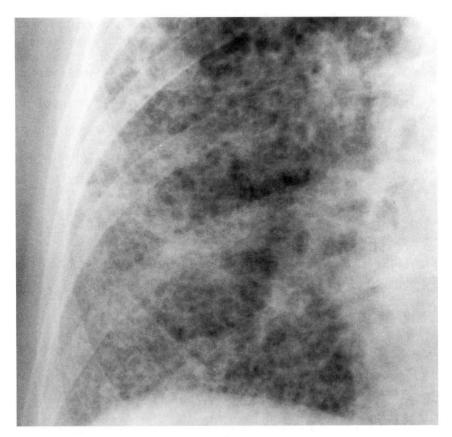

Figure 16 Diffuse reticulo-nodular shadowing in a case of fibrosing alveolitis

Cavitation

This usually occurs in nodular lesions. The commonest causes are tuberculosis, pneumonia (especially due to staphylococcus and klebsiella), primary peripheral bronchial carcinomas and pulmonary metastases. Abscess cavities are initially thickwalled, but with resolution of surrounding consolidation become smooth and thinner. Malignant cavities are often eccentric and have nodular, irregular margins.

Mediastinum

Mediastinal shift

The mediastinum may shift towards the side of collapse or fibrosis within the lung. Congenital lobar emphysema, tension pneumothorax or large pleural effusions will push the mediastinum to the contralateral side.

Mediastinal masses

The mediastinum is conveniently divided into three compartments. The *anterior* mediastinum lies anterior to the anterior surface of the pericardium and the trachea. The *middle* mediastinum includes the contents of the pericardium as well as the trachea. The *posterior* mediastinum lies behind the trachea and the posterior surface of the pericardium. Large mass lesions may lie in all three compartments. The aortic arch will also be present in all three parts of the mediastinum.

Common mediastinal mass lesions include:

1. *Anterior mediastinum*: lymph node enlargement; retrosternal goitre; thymoma. Look for tracheal deviation and narrowing.
2. *Middle mediastinum*: lymph node enlargement; aortic arch aneurysm; bronchogenic cyst; bronchogenic carcinoma.
3. *Posterior mediastinum*: hiatus hernia; oesophageal dilatation; aneurysm of descending aorta; neurogenic tumour; paravertebral mass.

CT and MRI are particularly helpful in determining the nature, location and extent of mediastinal masses.

3 Other Imaging Modalities

Ultrasound

Ultrasound scanning is a rapid and non-invasive method that can be performed at the bedside. The main applications of ultrasound are:

Chest

Assessing pleural and subphrenic disease. It will, for instance, differentiate pleural effusion from pleural thickening.

Abdomen

1. Suspected gallstones or cholecystitis.
2. Suspected liver metastases, although CT is more sensitive.
3. Jaundice or liver function tests with an obstructive pattern.
4. Pancreatitis, particularly to show or exclude gallstones and pseudocysts.
5. Possible aortic aneurysms, but CT is preferred for suspected leak or dissection.
6. Suspected abdominal sepsis. The subphrenic/subhepatic spaces and pelvis are well shown but ultrasond is less useful in mid-abdomen. If negative and clinical suspicion is high, use CT.
7. Guiding needle aspiration or drainage of fluid collections. Nephrostomies and cholecystostomies are also performed under ultrasound control.

Pelvis

1. Suspected pelvic masses.
2. Pelvic inflammatory disease or ectopic pregnancy.
3. Possible non-viable pregnancy.

Urinary Tract

1. Renal failure, although a normal scan does not always exclude obstruction.
2. Urinary tract infection in childhood.
3. Suspected renal mass.
4. Prostatic enlargement, to show upper tracts and bladder pre- and postvoiding.
5. Suspected scrotal mass and/or pain.

Vascular system

Colour Doppler ultrasound shows blood flow. As well as demonstrating venous patency or occlusion (see above), it is also helpful in evaluating arterial stenoses, for instance in the carotid artery.

Echocardiography accurately demonstrates pericardial effusions and valvular disease and, to some extent, myocardial function. Transoesophageal ultrasound is a useful method of demonstrating the presence or absence of aortic arch dissection.

Limitations

1. Distended bowel, for instance due to paralytic ileus, may cause image degradation.
2. Obesity may limit ultrasound transmission.
3. Abdominal incisions and tenderness may prevent good contact between the probe and skin surface.

Computed tomography

CT remains the optimal investigation for many problems within the head, chest and abdomen. It is the simplest method of staging most malignant diseases and monitoring their response to chemotherapy. CT provides valuable preoperative information about complex masses and is widely used for postoperative complications. It allows accurate guidance of needle aspiration, biopsies and drainage. CT also has an important role in evaluating trauma to the head and body.

There are several indications for CT.

Head

1. Following trauma, CT will answer the questions: (i) is there evidence of brain injury and (ii) is there evidence of intracranial haemorrhage or raised intracranial pressure?
2. Cerebrovascular accidents; CT will show the nature and the site of CVAs.
3. Suspected intracranial mass lesions; for example when cerebral metastases, primary brain tumour and brain abscesses are possibilities.

Chest

1. Diffuse lung disease. Thin section, high definition CT (HDCT)is sensitive in detecting and diagnosing the nature of diffuse lung disease; for example pulmonary fibrosis, emphysema and bronchiectasis.
2. Staging lung cancer and showing pulmonary metastases. A solitary nodule may be difficult to diagnose and needle biopsy may be required.
3. Pleural disease: CT may distinguish empyema from lung abscess,

demonstrate the extent of pleural tumours, distinguish between pleural fluid and thickening and demonstrate pleural plaques after asbestos exposure.

4. Mediastinal diseases: showing the extent of tumours and aortic arch abnormalities.

Contrast enhancement demonstrates pulmonary and systemic blood vessels. CT scanning is generally a rapid investigation. Most CT units have sufficient room to manage patients who arrive on beds with life-support and monitoring equipment. The bore of the CT gantry is sufficiently short and wide to allow good access to the patient during scanning. It should be remembered that CT scanning results in a comparatively high dose of irradiation.

Magnetic resonance imaging

MRI does not use ionizing radiation and it is now applicable in a wide range of clinical situations. The principal areas are the central nervous system, musculoskeletal system including the spine, oncology and the cardiovascular system.

In the chest, MRI will show morphological abnormalities of the heart and great vessels, giving haemodynamic information as well. MRI is also helpful in demonstrating mediastinal disease, particularly tumours and lymphadenopathy. It has a limited role in evaluating pulmonary disease and CT is generally superior in this regard.

Limitations

MRI is contraindicated in patients: with cardiac pacemakers, which will malfunction in the strong magnetic field; with ferromagnetic surgical clips, especially when these are applied to blood vessels; with loose ferromagnetic foreign bodies, for instance in the eyes. Standard monitoring and anaesthetic equipment should not be used in conjunction with patients undergoing MR imaging. However, non-magnetic anaesthetic machines are now available and monitoring may be performed beyond the magnetic field, using fibreoptic connections.

Radionuclide imaging

Although there are many clinical applications of radionuclide imaging, only ventilation and perfusion scanning of the lungs will be considered here. The main indication for lung scanning is the diagnosis of pulmonary embolism, but it is also used for the evaluation of emphysema.

Pulmonary ventilation scanning is usually performed with the isotopes of xenon or krypton, or technetium-labelled aerosols. ^{133}Xe is most commonly used, has a half-life of 5.7 days and may be used to assess areas of air trapping as well as areas of well-ventilated lungs. $^{81}Kr^m$ has a half-life of 13 seconds, depends on a cyclotron for its availability and is limited to defining ventilation. $^{99}Tc^m$ DTPA aerosol is convenient, readily available and cheap, but has the disadvantage of being deposited in major airways of patients with obstructive airways disease.

Perfusion scanning usually involves an intravenous injection of $^{99}Tc^m$ labelled albumen microspheres or microaggregates. Contraindications are pulmonary arterial hypertension and right-to-left cardiac shunts. The characteristic finding in pulmonary embolism is a perfusion defect corresponding to an identifiable segment or lobe without a matching ventilation defect. Matching ventilation and perfusion defects may be seen with a variety of pulmonary parenchymal abnormalities.

^{67}Gallium scanning has been used to evaluate granulomatous lung disease, especially sarcoid, occult infection, especially due to *Pneumocystis carinii*, and tumours.

Percutaneous lung biopsy

Percutaneous biopsy may involve a cutting needle or aspiration via a fine needle. Biopsy is contraindicated in patients on anticoagulants or with clotting diathesis and is inadvisable in patients with bullous emphysema or those who have had pneumonectomy. The patient's co-operation is required. Coughing is a further contraindication.

The diagnostic yield of fine needle aspiration (FNA) is approximately 90% for non-lymphomatous malignant lesions and 85% for benign lesions. Large-bore cutting needles are used for pleural based or very peripheral lung lesions, having ascertained by CT that the lesion is avascular in nature. Core biopsy is associated with a higher incidence of pneumothorax than is FNA. The incidence of pneumothorax is 15%, one-third of which require drainage. Biopsy is carried out using biplanar screening or CT.

Questions

Question 1

A 42 year old woman was given a general anaesthetic for removal of her wisdom teeth. Following the procedure, she developed surgical emphysema in her neck. This is the anteroposterior (AP) erect chest radiograph. What does it demonstrate? What is the management? What is the cause of this complication?

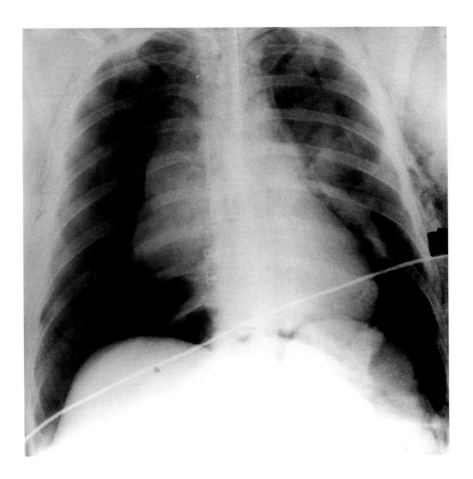

Question 2

This is the PA chest radiograph of an 81 year old woman. Apart from the slight rotation, describe the abnormalities. What is the cause?

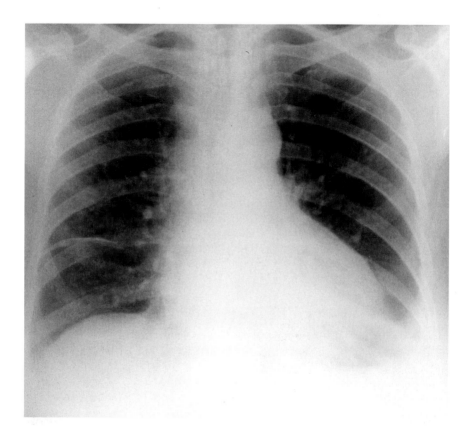

Question 3

This is the PA chest radiograph of a 47 year old woman admitted with acute onset of dyspnoea, fever and rightsided pleuritic chest pain. Describe the radiological signs. What are the likely causes?

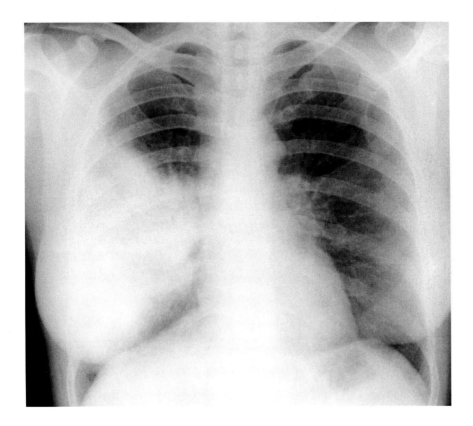

Question 4

This is the AP chest radiograph of a 76 year old woman with chronic respiratory impairment. Describe the abnormality and explain the cause of this appearance.

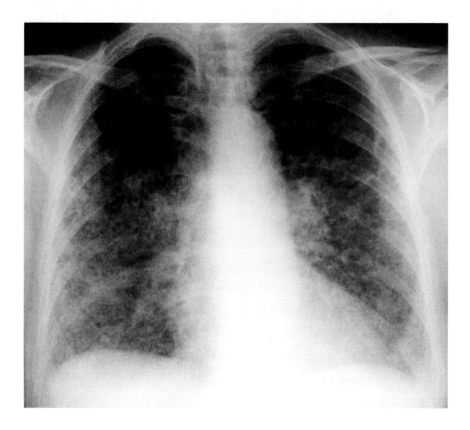

Question 5

This is a preoperative erect AP chest radiograph in a patient with dyspnoea. Describe the abnormalities.

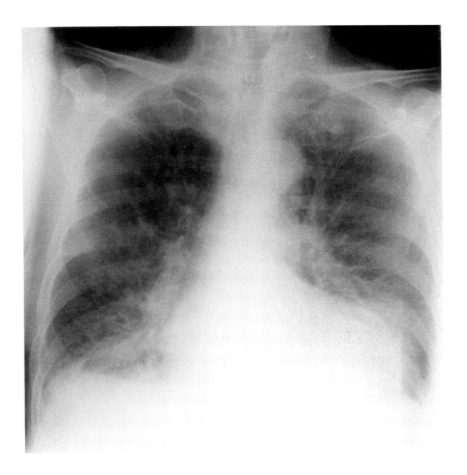

Question 6

This supine chest radiograph of a 67 year old man was taken on arrival at the Intensive Care Unit following an elective graft repair of an abdominal aortic aneurysm. The preoperative chest radiograph was clear. The patient did not aspirate during the procedure and is not uraemic. What is the cause of the radiological abnormality? How would you manage this case?

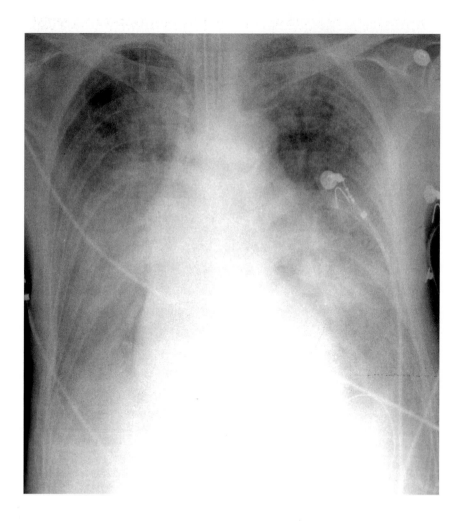

Question 7

This is the erect PA chest radiograph of a 57 year old man with longstanding dyspnoea. Describe the radiological signs. What is the most likely cause? What precautions should be taken if this patient is given a general anaesthetic?

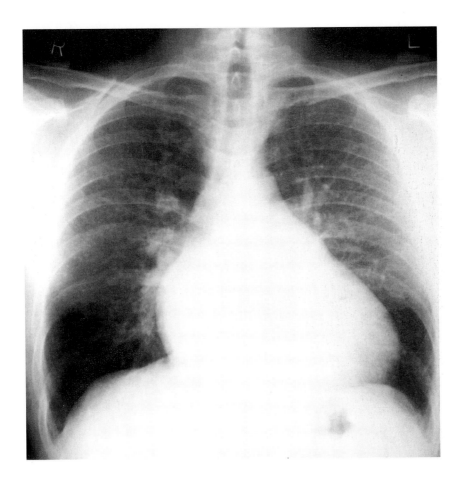

Question 8

This is a normal venogram study. What are the labelled structures 1–6?

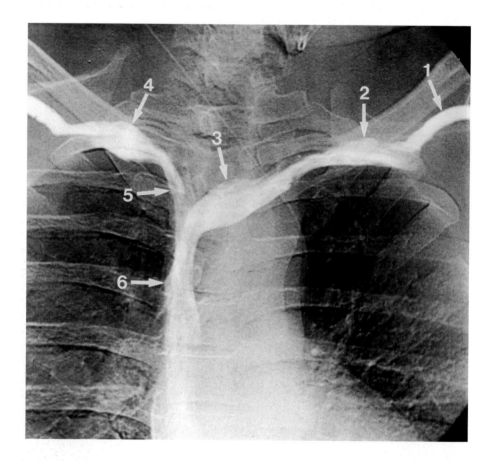

Question 9

This is the supine chest radiograph of a 35 year old patient who, six days previously, was involved in a house fire and suffered 34% body surface area burns. Describe the abnormalities. What condition is the patient most likely to be suffering from? What are the other possible causes?

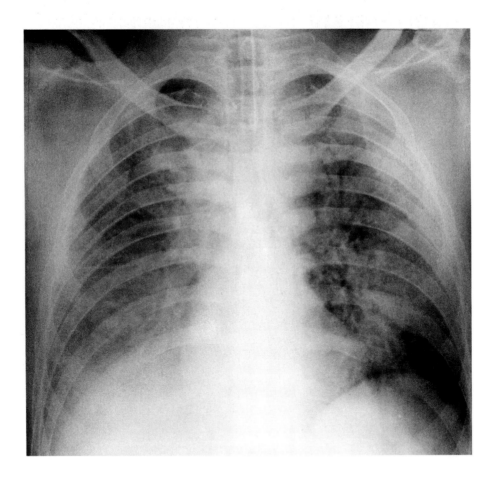

Question 10

This 32 year old male insulin-dependent diabetic has been troubled with a cough. Describe the abnormalities on the posteroanterior chest radiograph. What is the diagnosis?

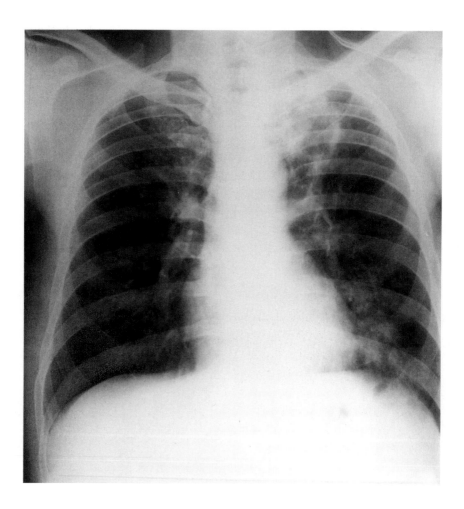

Question 11

A 28 year old man presented with a cough, fever, dyspnoea, arthralgia and malaise. He also complained of eye problems and a skin rash. Describe the abnormalities on this chest radiograph. What is the diagnosis?

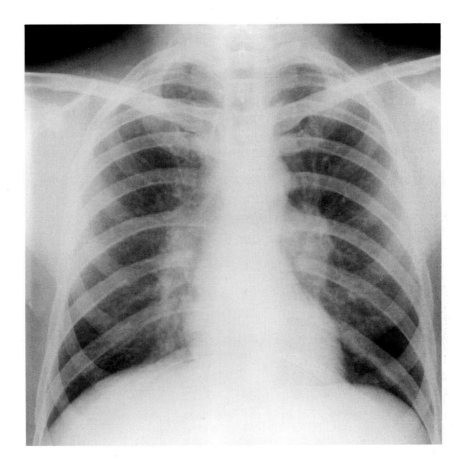

Question 12

A 65 year old male patient is ventilated on the intensive care unit for respiratory failure following a cholecystectomy seven days previously. He has a raised white cell count of $19 \times 10^9/l$ and a temperature of 38°C. This figure demonstrates two images of an ultrasound scan of his right upper quadrant in the sagittal plane. What abnormality do these images demonstrate and what is its management?

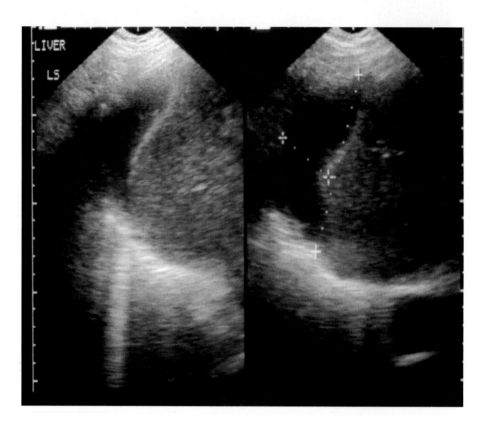

Question 13

This is the PA chest radiograph of a 28 year old asymptomatic woman. Describe the abnormalities and give the management for elective surgery.

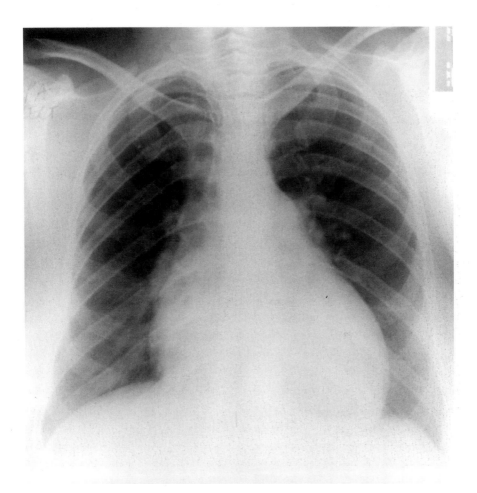

Question 14

This is the AP chest radiograph of a 61 year old man due for elective surgery who at the present time has an exacerbation of his condition. Describe the radiological signs.

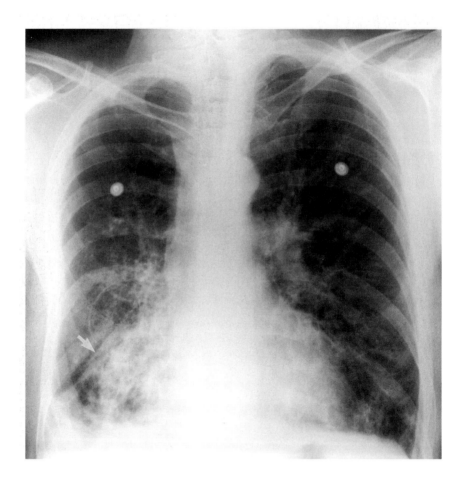

Question 15

This is the posteroanterior chest radiograph of a 74 year old man with longstanding dyspnoea. What are the radiological features and diagnosis?

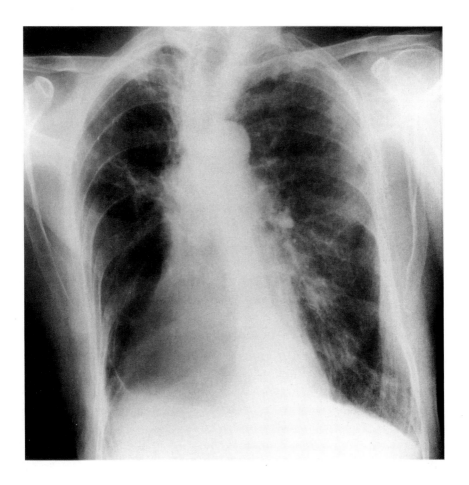

Question 16

This is a supine chest radiograph of a 22 year old female taken at day 3 postpartum. She developed respiratory problems requiring ventilation. What are structures 1–4 and what are their acceptable positions on a chest radiograph? Describe the radiological features and give the diagnosis

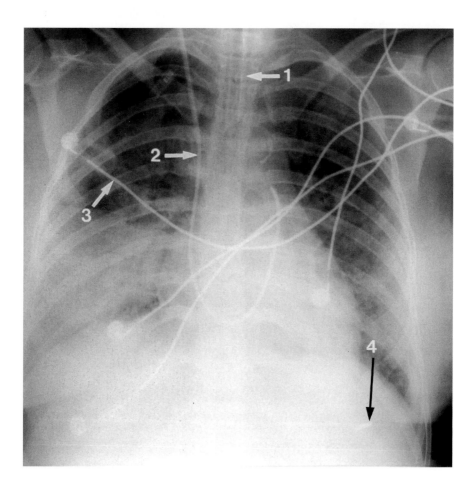

Question 17

A 47 year old woman in the Intensive Care Unit with adult respiratory distress syndrome has had a leftsided subclavian central line inserted. The postinsertion supine chest radiograph is shown. What is the abnormality and what is the treatment?

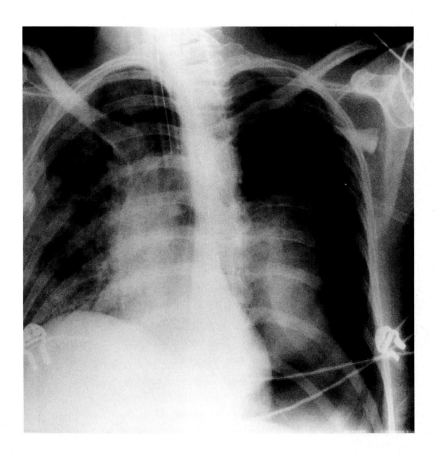

Question 18

This edge-enhanced occipitofrontal radiograph of the skull of a nine month old was taken when a bruise was noted on the head. What is the radiological sign? What diagnosis should be considered and what further investigations are necessary?

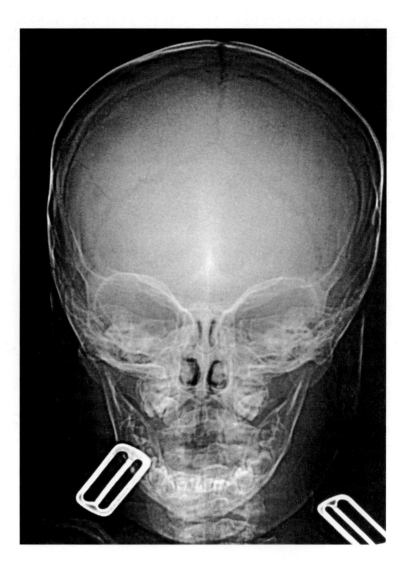

Question 19

This is the preoperative posteroanterior chest radiograph of a 57 year old woman, who has no chest complaints and has not been involved in previous trauma. What are the radiological features and diagnosis?

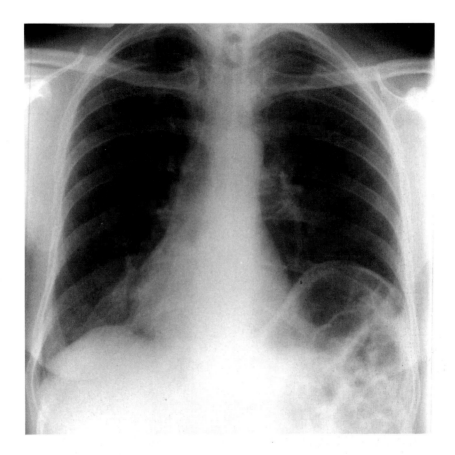

Question 20

This is the preoperative posteroanterior chest radiograph of a 26 year old man. He has no history of chest disease and has no signs or symptoms related to his chest. Describe the abnormalities. What are their causes?

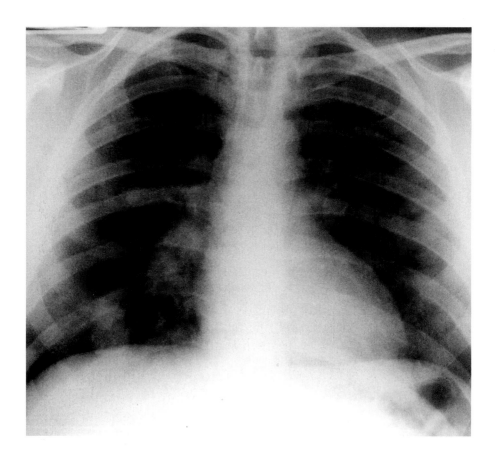

Question 21

A 64 year old retired miner had this PA chest radiograph taken because of increasing dyspnoea. The radiological appearances had not changed since a chest radiograph six months previously. What are the radiological signs and what are the diagnoses?

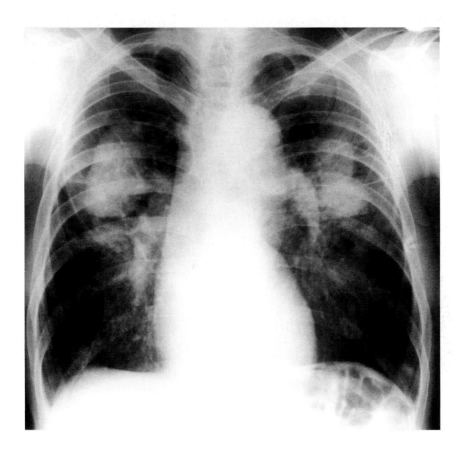

Question 22

This is the slightly rotated preoperative posteroanterior chest radiograph of a 66 year old woman. What abnormality is demonstrated? What are the possible complications?

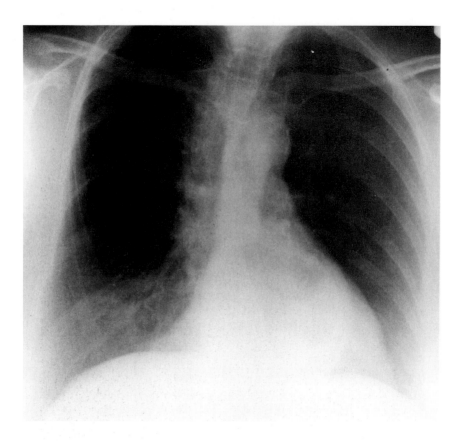

Question 23

This is the lateral cervical spine view taken, with the head in the vertical position on a 24 year old male with an earring who sustained head and neck injuries following a motor vehicle accident. What are the structures indicated by arrows 1–10? What is the radiological diagnosis and short- term management?

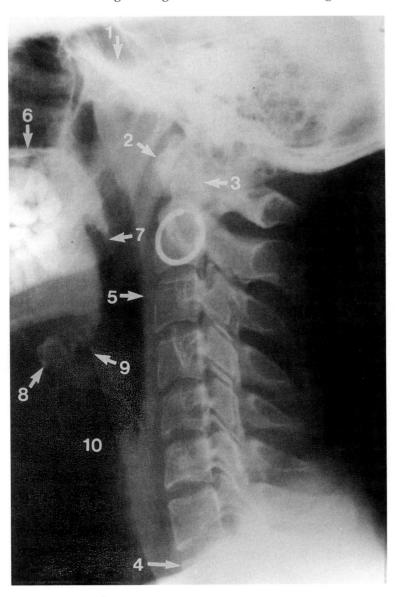

Question 24

This is the slightly rotated supine chest radiograph of a 26 year old male asthmatic and heroin addict who is being ventilated for his respiratory failure. What radiological abnormalities are demonstrated and how would you manage this case?

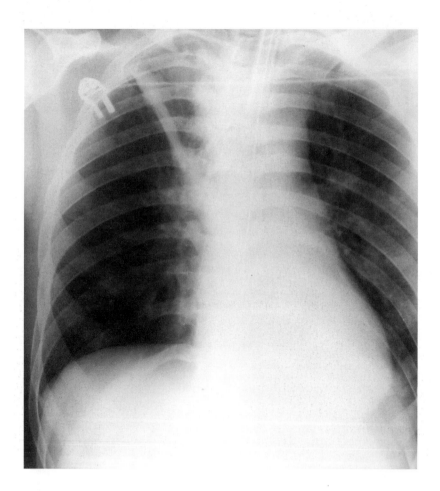

Question 25

This is the posteroanterior chest radiograph of a 72 year old woman with weight loss. Describe the radiological abnormalities. What are the diagnoses?

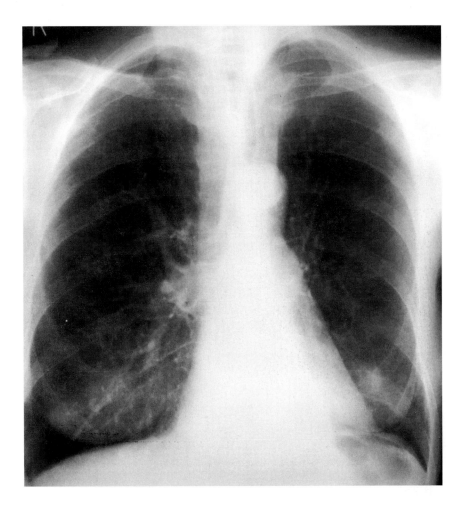

Question 26

This 55 year old female complains of haemoptysis. What are the radiological features and their anatomical site?

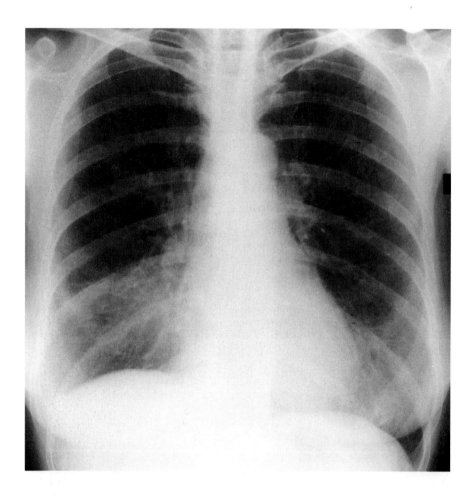

Question 27

This is the supine chest radiograph of a 17 year old methadone addict who required ventilatory support following aspiration of vomit. Describe the abnormalities. How would you manage this case?

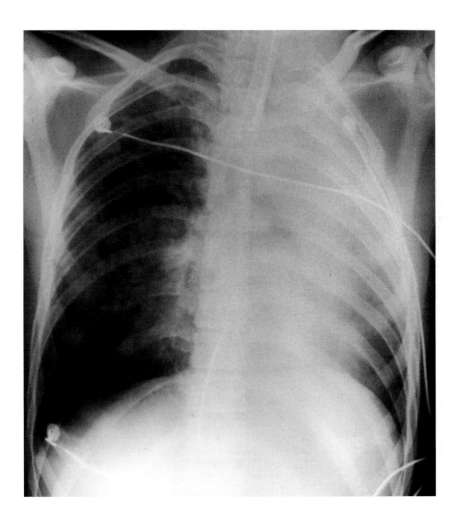

Question 28

This is a preoperative chest radiograph of a 64 year old woman. Ignore the overlying buttons. What abnormality is demonstrated and how does this relate to a general anaesthetic?

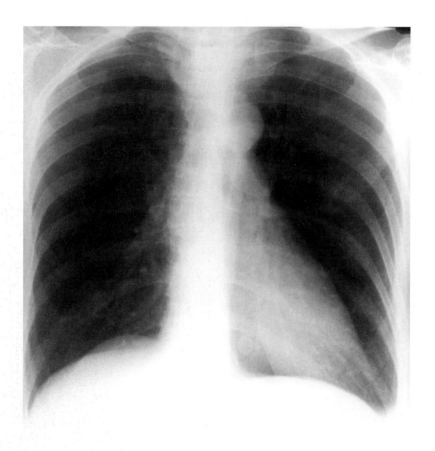

Question 29

A 32 year old woman was a pedestrian involved in a collision with a motor vehicle. This portable semisupine AP radiograph was taken in the emergency room, soon after admission. What abnormality is demonstrated? What is its significance?

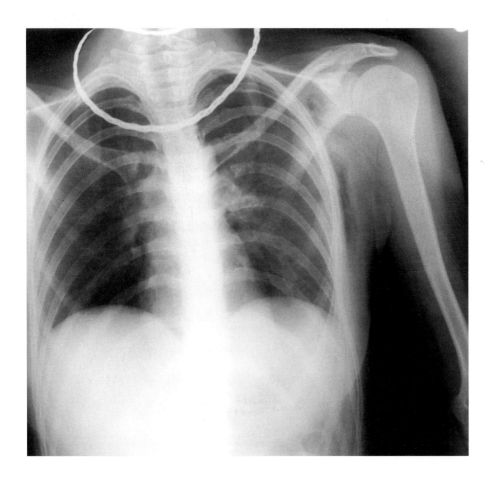

Question 30

A 27 year old man sustained fractures of his pelvis and femur in a motor vehicle accident and was admitted to an orthopaedic ward; 24 hours later he developed respiratory problems. This is his supine chest radiograph following endotracheal intubation and insertion of a central line, a Swan– Ganz catheter and a nasogastric tube. Describe the radiological abnormalities. What is the diagnosis?

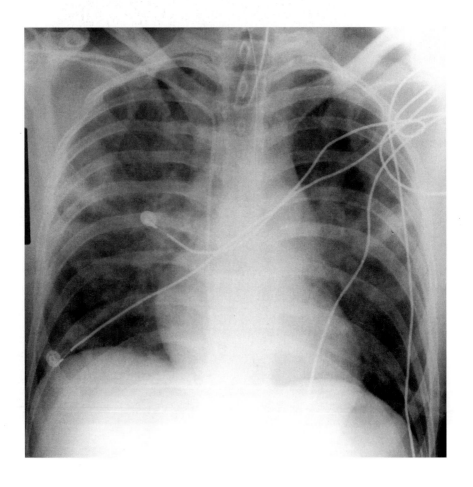

Question 31

This is a preoperative chest radiograph. Describe the radiological signs. What is the diagnosis?

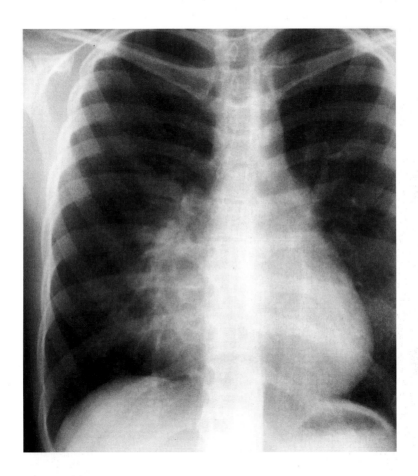

Question 32

AP and lateral radiographs of a 17 year old female involved in a motor vehicle accident. What are the radiological signs and diagnosis? Is this injury stable or unstable? What is the required management?

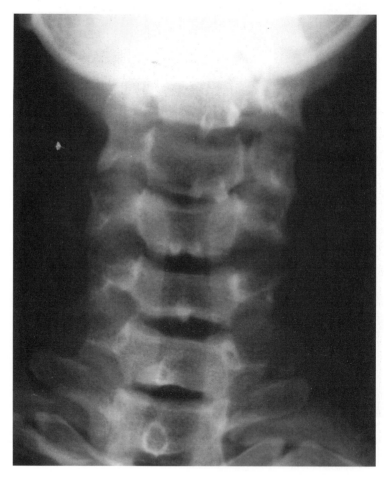

AP Radiograph

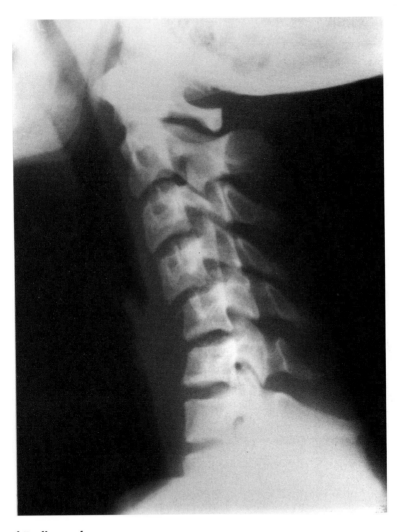

Lateral Radiograph

Question 33

This is the supine chest radiograph of a 29 year old man taken on the second day following ventilation. The patient was intubated because of respiratory failure due to acute smoke inhalation and 40% body surface area burns. What other abnormality is demonstrated and what is the management?

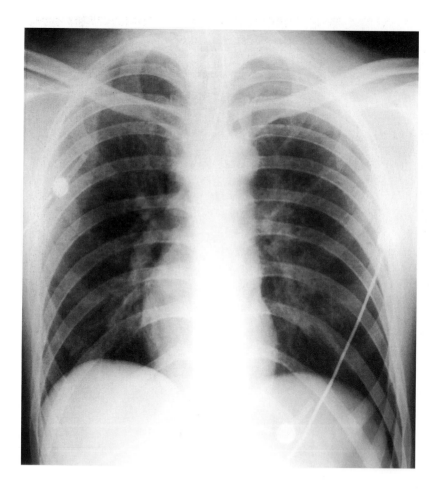

Question 34

This 84 year old woman was admitted with severe abdominal pain and vomiting. This chest radiograph was taken at the time. What is the abnormality shown and what is its significance?

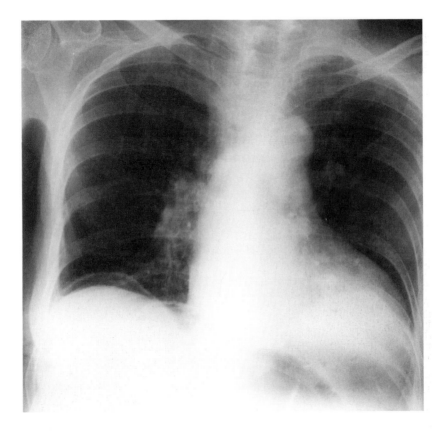

Question 35

This is the anteroposterior chest radiograph of a 59 year old man with gastric outlet obstruction. Describe the abnormalities. What is the diagnosis?

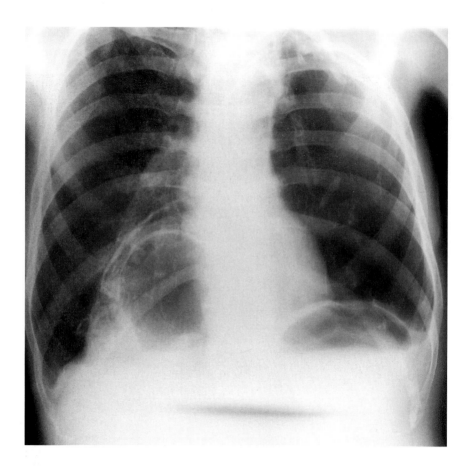

Question 36

A 46 year old woman with acute myeloid leukaemia has had a Hickman line for 15 weeks, without complications from the line. This patient has received a bone marrow transplant and is immunosuppressed. She has been dyspnoeic for some time but has become acutely unwell. Describe the radiological abnormalities and give their cause.

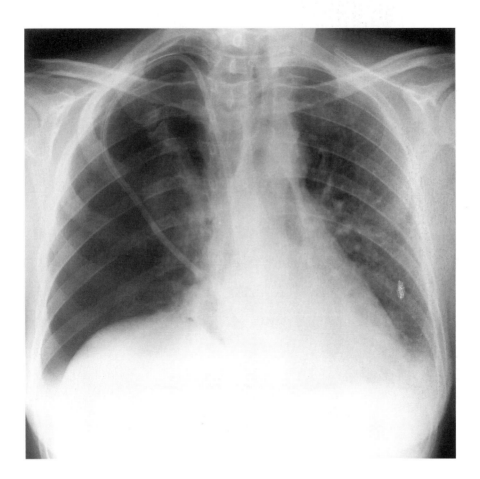

Question 37

A 71 year old man with a history of asbestos exposure presents with haemoptysis. This is his PA chest radiograph. Describe the abnormalities and give the diagnosis.

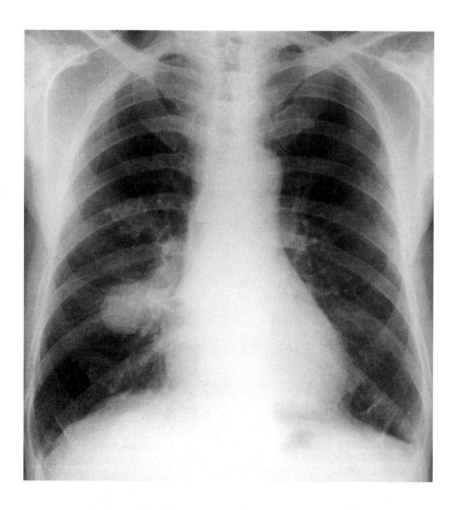

Question 38

This barium swallow, shown here in the lateral projection, was performed on a 94 year old woman. A recent chest radiograph had shown consolidation of the right lung base. What is the abnormality?

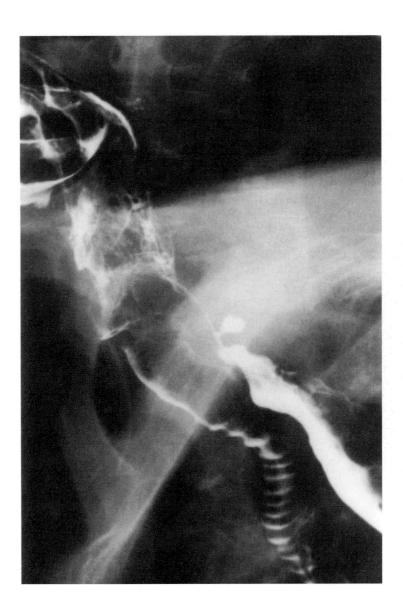

Question 39

This is the CT brain scan of a 62 year old man with a three week history of leftsided weakness. There has been sudden deterioration in this patient's symptoms. What are the structures numbered 1–8?

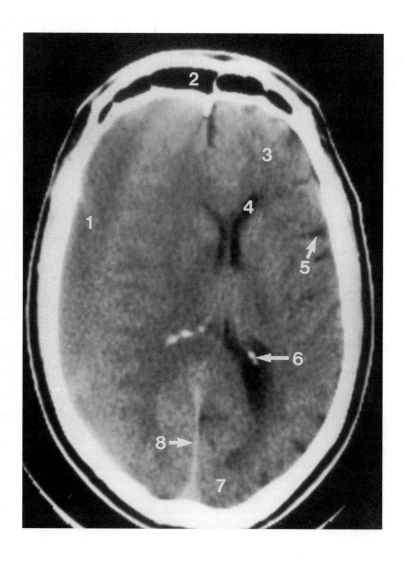

Question 40

This is the chest radiograph of a tachypnoeic 16 hour old baby who had been delivered by caesarean section. What is the diagnosis?

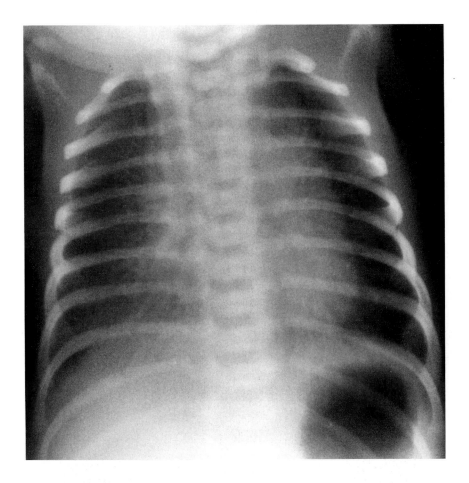

Question 41

This is the supine chest radiograph of a 48 year old man taken four days after a home fire in which he suffered acute inhalation injury and 24% body surface area burns. He has a raised temperature and white cell count. Ignore an overlying lead. Describe the chest radiograph abnormalities. What diagnosis should be considered? What are the risk factors and the diagnostic procedure of choice?

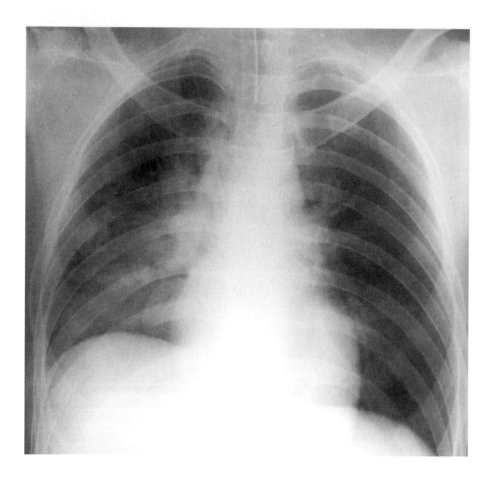

Question 42

A lateral cervical radiograph of an 18 month old baby who sustained head and neck injuries in a motor vehicle accident. What are the radiological signs? What is the management?

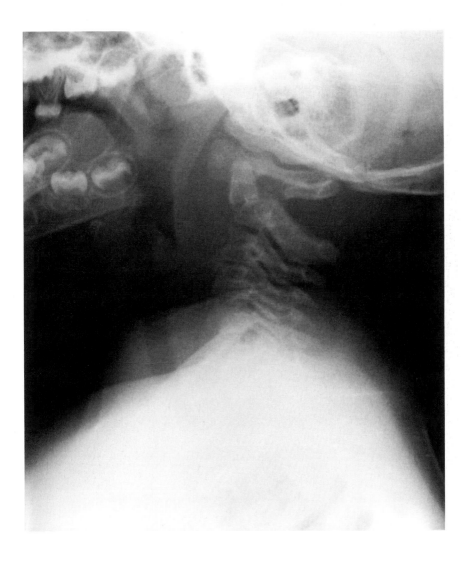

Question 43

A 38 year old drunken woman fell down a flight of stairs and sustained an injury to the left side of her chest. On examination there is asymmetrical expansion of her chest. This slightly rotated AP supine chest radiograph was taken in the Accident and Emergency department. The arrows point to posterior rib fractures. What other abnormalities are present and how would you manage this case?

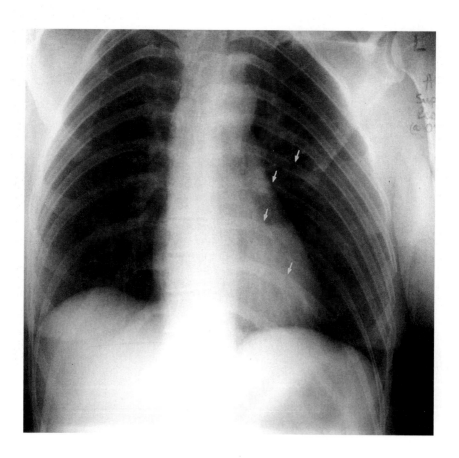

Question 44

This is the supine chest radiograph of a 36 hour old premature neonate with respiratory difficulties. Describe the abnormalities and your management.

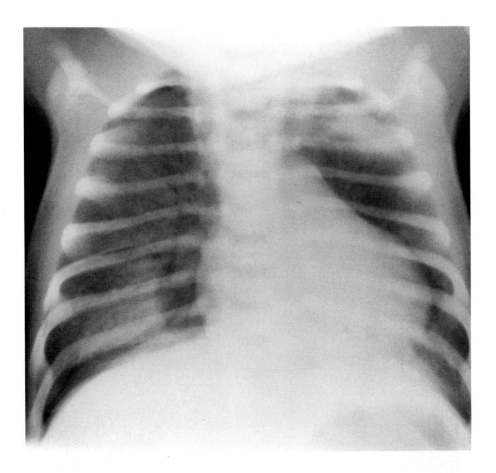

Question 45

This is a lateral cervical radiograph of a 63 year old man. Describe the major abnormality. What are the problems and solutions of a general anaesthetic?

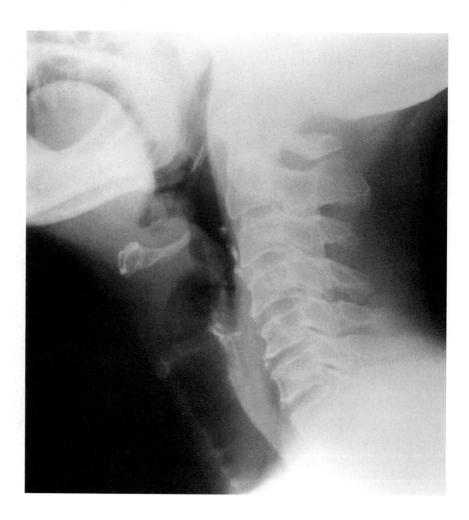

Question 46

This is the posteroanterior chest radiograph of a 40 year old man with poly-cythaemia, who presented with dyspnoea and pleuritic chest pain. What abnormalities are demonstrated and how would you manage this case?

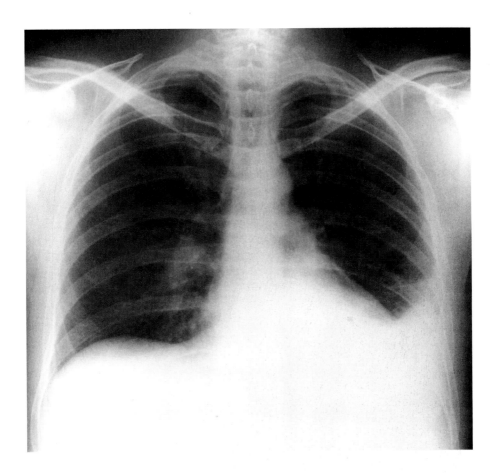

Question 47

This is the supine chest radiograph of a 62 year old taken on the intensive care unit after a coronary artery bypass graft operation. Describe the abnormalities and how you would manage this case.

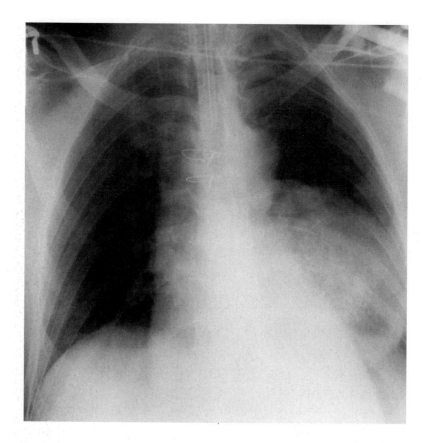

Question 48

This is the preoperative chest and abdominal film of a 11 year old male patient. What abnormalities are demonstrated? Discuss the physiology and give the management.

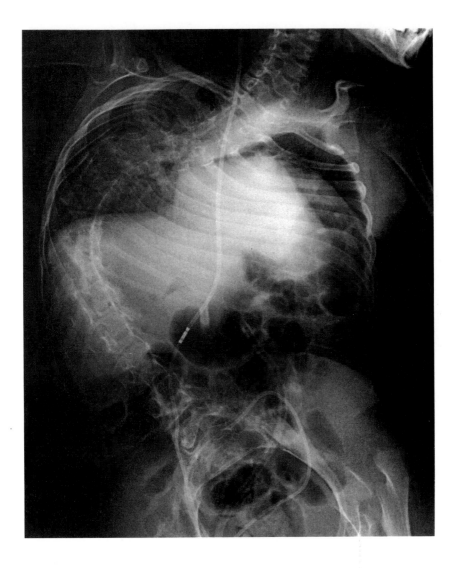

Question 49

Coronal CT is performed in cases of facial trauma to assess the extent of facial bone fractures. This is one such image of a 24 year old male involved in a motor vehicle accident. Describe the findings and discuss the management.

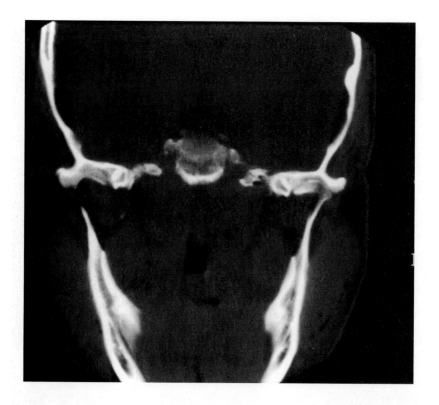

Question 50

This is the rotated AP chest radiograph of a 78 year old woman following a procedure on the ward. What abnormalities are demonstrated and what is the management?

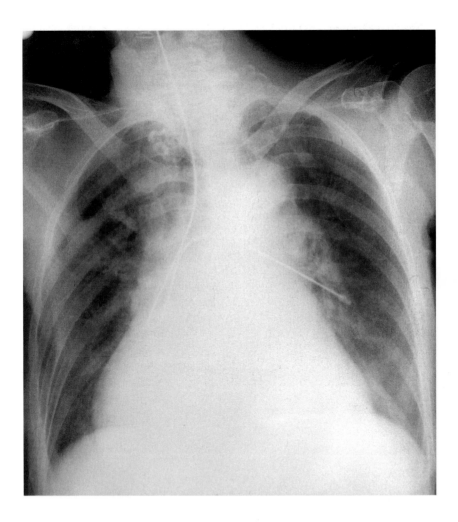

Question 51

This is the supine chest radiograph of a 20 year old male who sustained severe head injuries following a motor vehicle accident. A tracheostomy and the insertion of the tracheostomy tube were performed prior to the radiograph. What abnormalities are demonstrated and what is their significance?

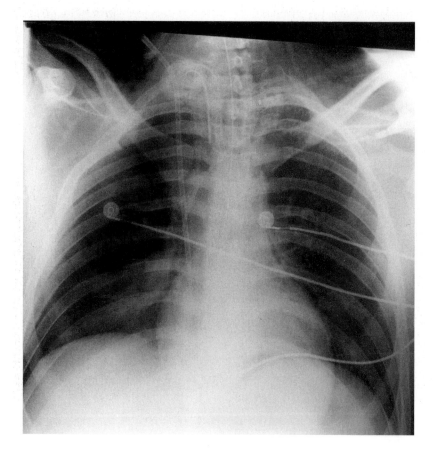

Question 52

A four year old boy who has been playing at a friend's house is brought into the Accident and Emergency Department with sudden onset of dyspnoea. This is one of two posteroanterior chest radiographs. What is the diagnosis?

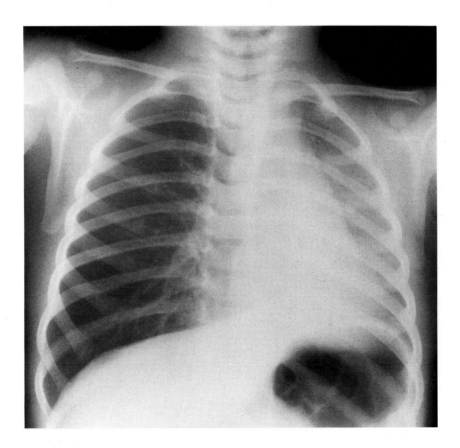

Question 53

This is an image from an intravascular contrast medium study in a 44 year old woman, following the injection of contrast medium via a catheter with its tip in the left subclavian vein. What does it demonstrate? What is the cause?

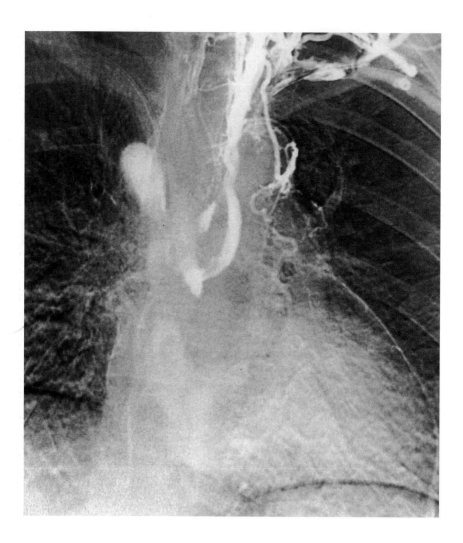

Question 54

This supine chest radiograph was taken after the insertion of a central line in a 42 year old ventilated patient. What abnormality is seen and what would be your management?

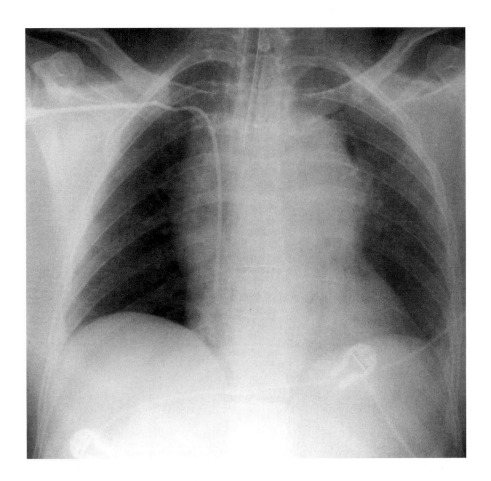

Question 55

This is the lateral radiograph of the sternum of a 32 year old man involved in a motor vehicle accident. What abnormality is demonstrated and what is the significance?

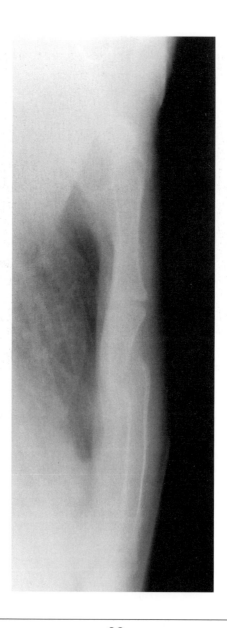

Question 56

A 41 year old man sustained an injury to the right side of his thorax in a motor vehicle accident. Three weeks later he was expectorating green sputum, had a temperature of 38°C and a white cell count of 19x10⁹/l. A PA chest radiograph was taken at this time. What does it demonstrate and what is the significance?

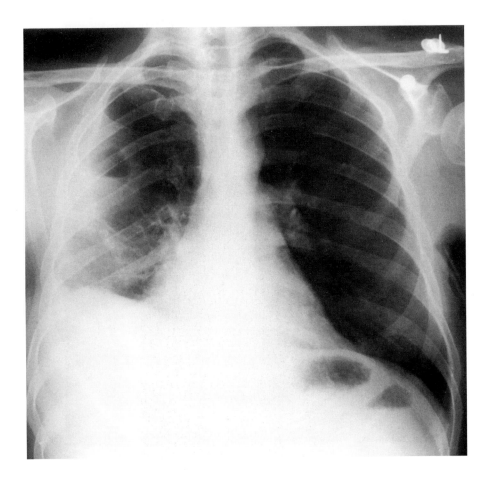

Question 57

This is an image from the CT brain scan of a 20 year old who is rapidly losing consciousness following a motor vehicle accident. Describe the abnormalities. What is the next management decision?

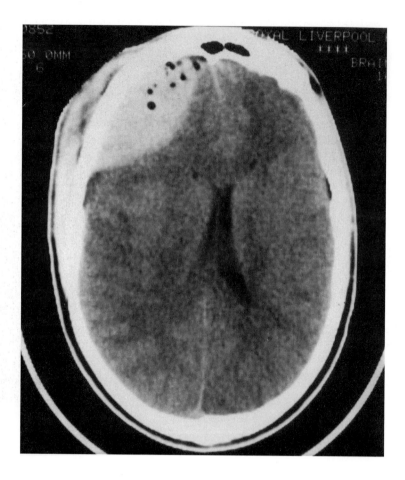

Question 58

This is the posteroanterior chest radiograph of a 53 year old man who had coronary artery bypass surgery nine weeks previously. Describe the abnormalities and suggest the cause and management.

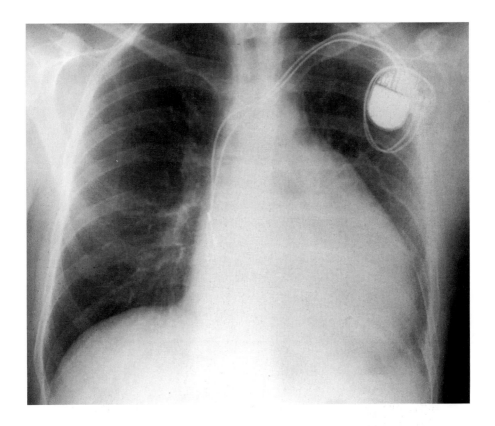

Question 59

This is the anteroposterior chest radiograph of a dyspnoeic 63 year old woman who has breast carcinoma. There is no history of cardiovascular disease and the chest radiograph one year previously was normal. Describe the abnormalities. What is the cause?

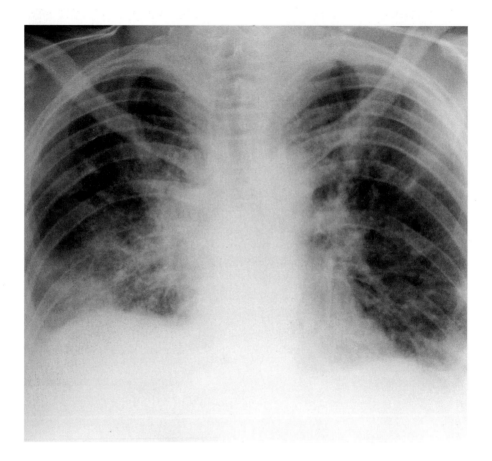

Question 60

This is the supine chest radiograph of a child who requires mechanical ventilation following near drowning. What abnormalities are shown? What is the management?

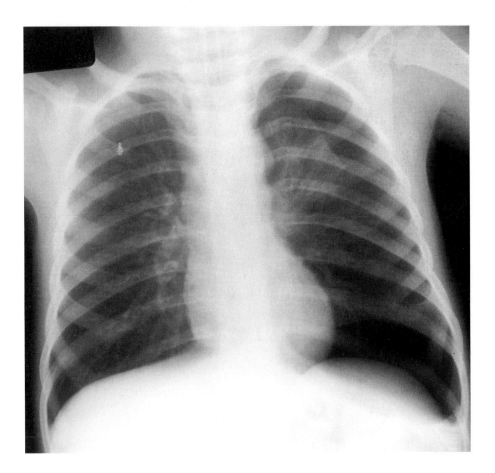

Question 61

This is the supine chest radiograph of a full-term baby who had fetal distress and now has respiratory distress. Which disease process do you suspect and what is your management?

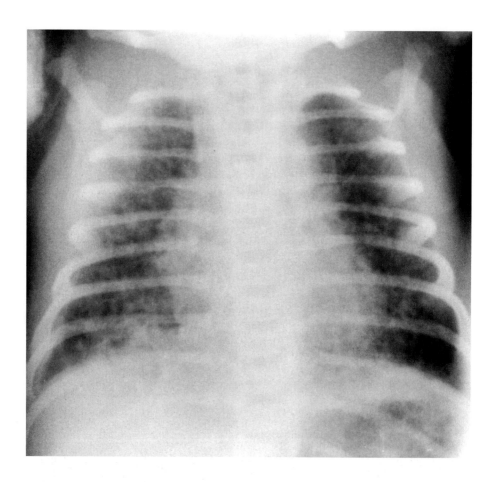

Question 62

A 68 year old man was admitted to the Accident and Emergency Department with a sudden onset of low back pain. This is his admission supine abdominal radiograph. What are the radiographic features and their significance? What is the management?

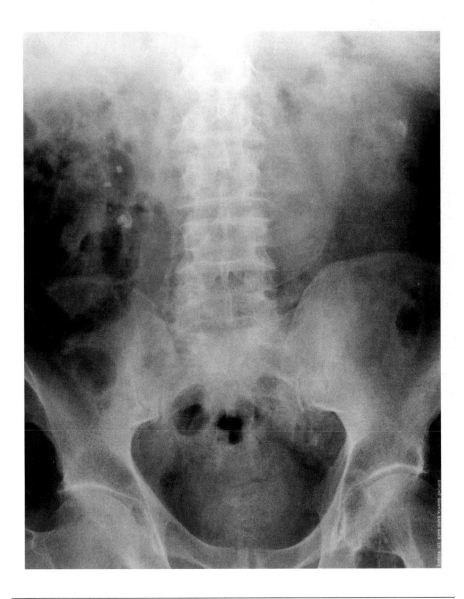

Question 63

This is a preoperative chest radiograph of a 74 year old man. What abnormality is present? What question would you ask the patient? What is the management?

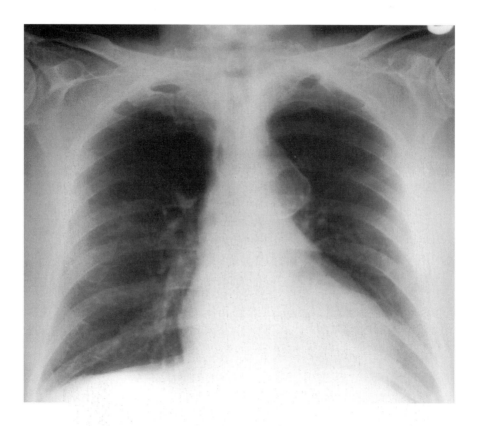

Question 64

An unenhanced CT scan of the head of a 33 year old woman who became unconscious following 36 hours of flu-like symptoms. What are the abnormal features and diagnosis? What further radiological investigation is required? What complication of this disease should be considered?

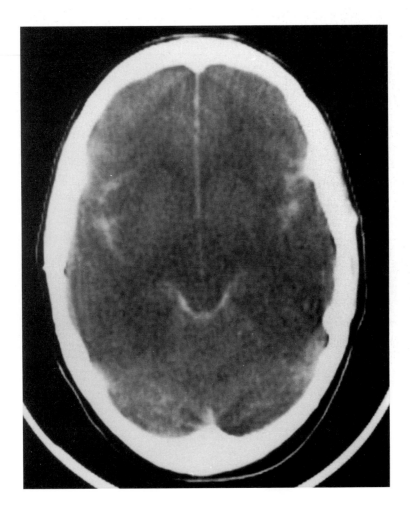

Question 65

A three month old baby was admitted with a clinical diagnosis of bronchiolitis. The admission chest radiograph showed bilateral overinflation of the lungs, indicating air trapping. On the second day following admission, the baby required ventilation because of progressive respiratory problems. This chest radiograph followed endotracheal intubation. Describe the radiological abnormalities. What is the diagnosis?

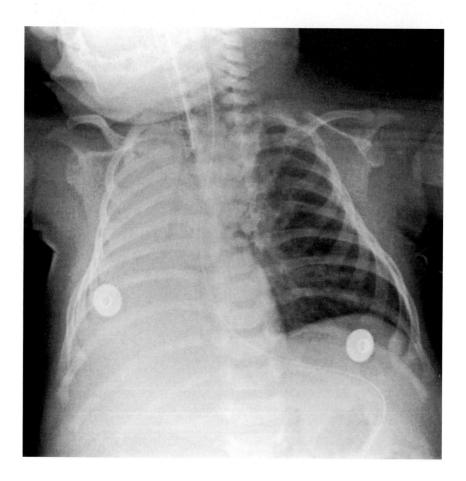

Question 66

This is the slightly rotated PA chest radiograph of a 43 year old woman receiving therapy through her long line. Prior to her therapy she had a normal chest radiograph. What is the significance of the abnormalities demonstrated?

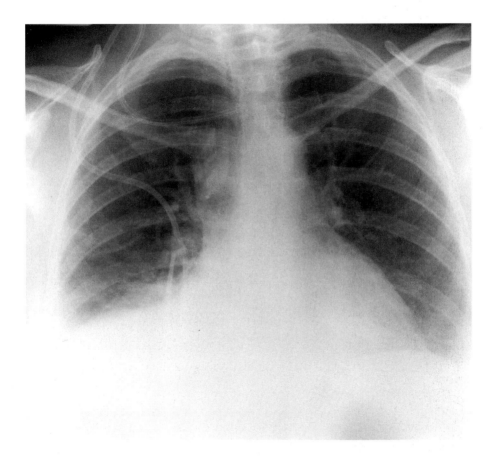

Question 67

This is the preoperative flexion lateral cervical spine radiograph of a 46 year old female. What radiological abnormality is demonstrated? What is the most likely cause in this case and what are the other possible causes of this condition? What is the management?

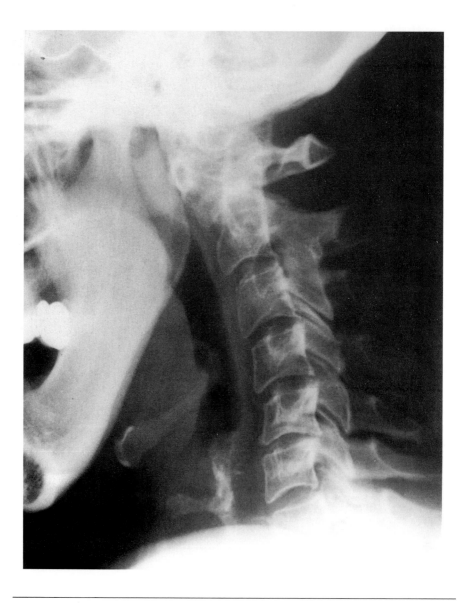

Question 68

This is the chest radiograph of a 38 year old man who was complaining of dyspnoea and leftsided pleuritic pain. Five weeks previously he had sustained upper abdominal injuries and rib fractures in a motor vehicle accident. What are the diagnosis and management?

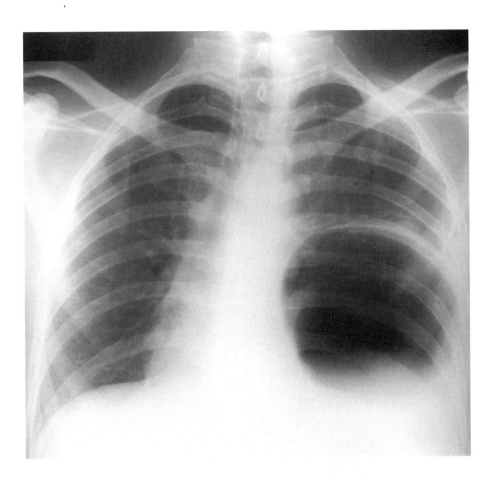

Question 69

An 80 year old lady presented to the Accident and Emergency Department with severe chest pain, dyspnoea and evidence of the superior vena caval syndrome. This is her admission chest radiograph. Describe the abnormality and give the diagnosis.

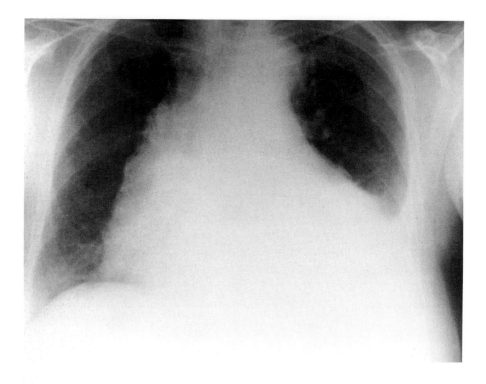

Question 70

A 50 year old male patient required ventilatory support following a stabbing injury to his abdomen and major surgery. This is a chest radiograph taken on the fifth day of his intensive care unit admission. Describe the abnormalities and their significance. How would you manage this case?

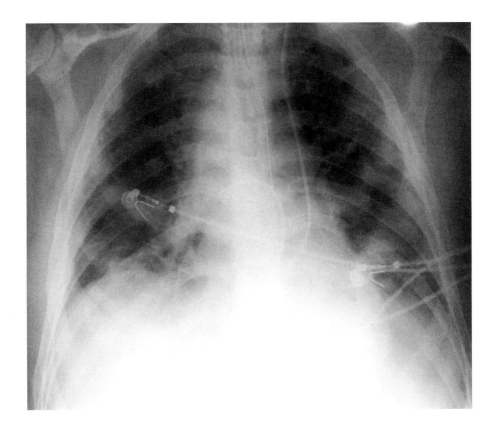

Question 71

This 52 year old man was admitted to the Accident and Emergency Department with vomiting and central abdominal pain radiating to the back. On examination he was hypotensive, had a generally tender abdomen and bruising of his loins. A plain abdominal radiograph demonstrated a gasless abdomen. A CT image of this man's abdomen is shown. What does it demonstrate and what are the prognostic indicators of this disease?

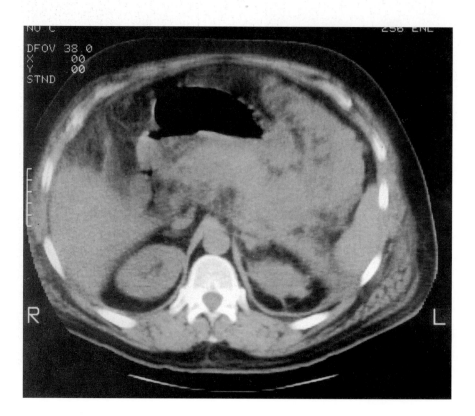

Question 72

This is the supine chest radiograph of a 28 year old man following a fall of 30 metres. Describe the radiological abnormalities and further management.

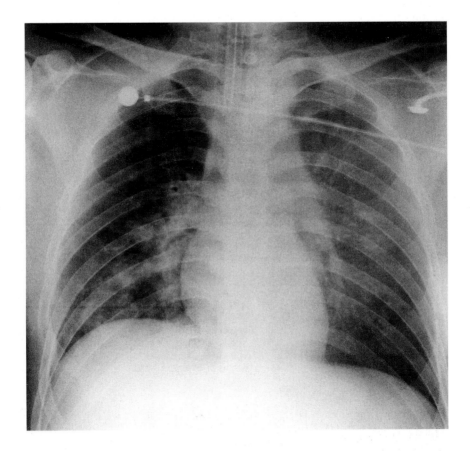

Question 73

This is the supine chest radiograph of a 57 year old immediately after long line insertion. A chest radiograph prior to this procedure was normal. What is the significance of the abnormality and what is the management?

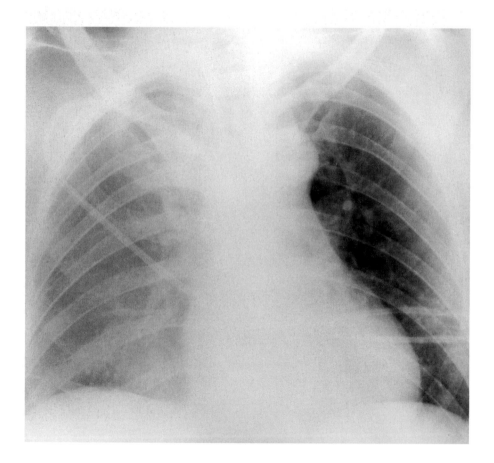

Question 74

This baby with hyaline membrane disease has deteriorating blood gases. Describe the abnormality and management.

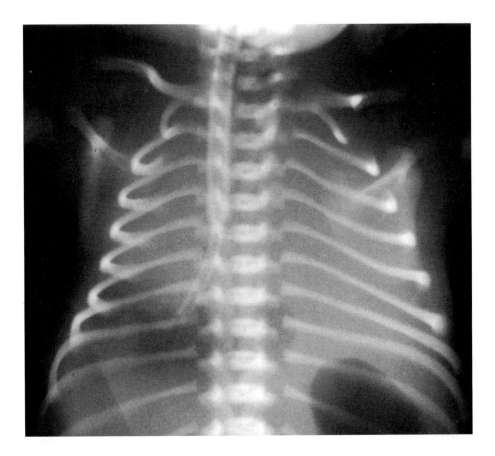

Question 75

This is the supine chest radiograph of a 32 year old woman with sickle cell anaemia whose normal haemoglobin is 7g/dl. She required ventilatory support following an episode of transfusion-induced reverse sequestration leading to a haemoglobin level of 12.4g/dl. What is the significance of the abnormalities and what is the management?

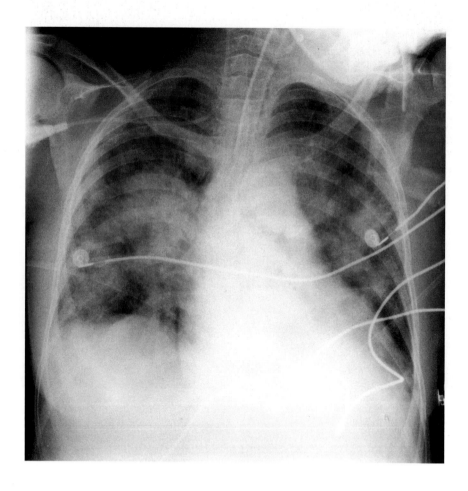

Question 76

This is an erect anteroposterior chest radiograph of a 78 year old man taken three hours after a barium swallow. The central line is in the normal position. What is the significance of the abnormalities demonstrated?

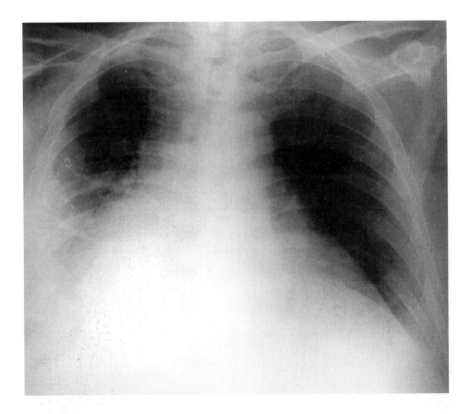

Question 77

This 21 year old man was involved in a motor vehicle accident. Describe the radiological abnormalities and give the underlying diagnosis and management.

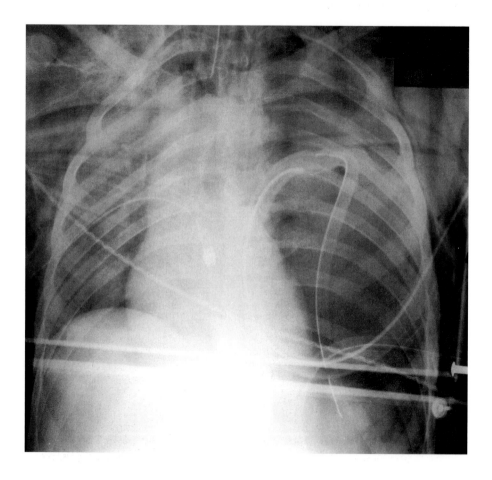

Question 78

This 69 year old man required ventilatory support following extensive surgery for carcinoma of the tongue. His preoperative chest radiograph was normal. A considerable amount of fluid was oozing from his wounds. This supine chest radiograph was taken four days after surgery. Describe the abnormalities and their significance.

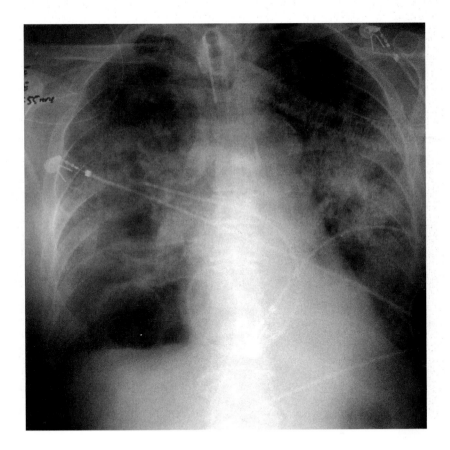

Question 79

A 47 year old woman required ventilation to treat her adult respiratory distress syndrome following major abdominal surgery. Her blood gases were deteriorating and this supine, slightly rotated chest radiograph was taken. What are the radiological abnormalities and how would you manage this case?

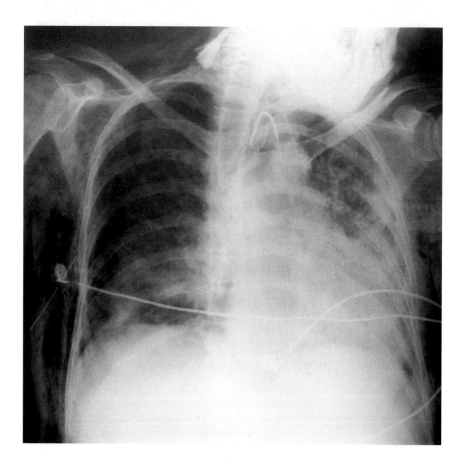

Question 80

This ventilated two day old baby's blood gases are deteriorating. Describe the abnormalities and the management in this case.

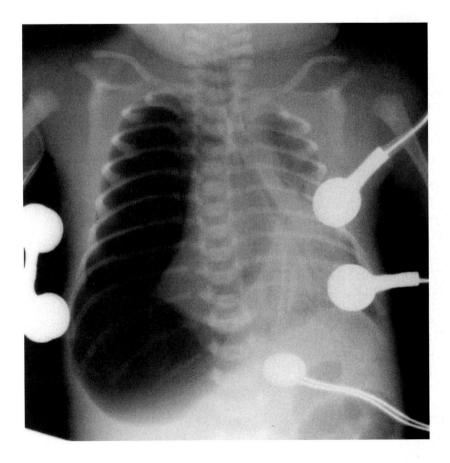

Answers

Answer 1

There are bilateral pneumothoraces with almost total collapse of both lungs, as demonstrated by large radiolucent pleural spaces devoid of vessels and the identification of the visceral pleural lines. There is also a pneumomediastinum, as demonstrated by a radiolucent region of air adjacent to the left heart border and aortic arch. Surgical emphysema with air present in the fascial planes and subcutaneous tissue within the neck and chest wall. The endotracheal tube is deviated to the left, indicating that there is higher pressure in the right hemithorax than the left. A monitor wire crosses over the thorax. The patient requires urgent insertion of bilateral chest drains, starting with the one on the right.

These pneumothoraces are iatrogenic and there are two theoretical mechanisms:

1. Abrasions of the mucosa of the pharynx, larynx or trachea followed by high pressure of the inhaled gases can produce surgical emphysema. The gases spread through the fascial planes to the neck and thoracic wall as well as to the mediastinum and pleural spaces.
2. Gas ruptures through the surface of the alveoli into the pulmonary interstitium and progresses centrally along blood vessels to the hilum. It then enters the pleural space and mediastinum, spreading into the fascial planes of the neck and thoracic wall. An initial high pressure is apparently required for this, although lower pressures will perpetuate the rupture.

Answer 2

The heart is moderately enlarged (cardiothoracic ratio 54%). There is blunting of both costophrenic angles, with a meniscus-shaped homogeneous density in the left costophrenic angle and obliteration of the left hemidiaphragm. These are the appearances of pleural effusions. On the right side, the horizontal fissure is filled with fluid. The cause in this case is likely to be congestive cardiac failure.

A small pleural effusion (less than 5ml) may be missed on the erect chest radiograph. As the volume increases, blunting of the posterior and lateral costophrenic angles occurs and homogeneous opacification of the lower chest develops with obliteration of the normal interface between aerated lung and hemidiaphragm. When the pleural effusion is large, fluid can be identified above the upper lobe apex. On the supine chest radiograph a unilateral pleural effusion will collect in the posterior pleural space, causing unilateral homogeneous opacification of that hemithorax. The pleural effusion in a supine radiograph can be confirmed by a radiograph taken with the patient in the lateral decubitus or erect position. The contour of free-running pleural fluid will then be identified. In patients who cannot be moved, an ultrasound scan will confirm the presence of a pleural effusion.

Answer 3

There is consolidation involving the right middle and lower zones. An air bronchogram is demonstrated adjacent to the right hilum. The consolidation is affecting the right upper and lower lobes. The most usual cause of this appearance in this clinical context is streptococcal or mycoplasma pneumonia; in this case it was due to *Legionella pneumophila*. The infective causes of lobar pneumonia are bacteria, tuberculosis, mycoplasma, fungi and viruses.

Consolidation, or air space shadowing, is caused by air in the lung being replaced by fluid (oedema), pus (pneumonia), blood (haemorrhage) or tumour cells. The smallest air space unit identifiable is the acinar nodule (4–10 mm diameter) which, when its air is replaced, has ill-defined margins. As adjacent acini become affected coalescence and homogeneous opacification are seen. Air bronchograms are identified when consolidated lung is adjacent to an air-containing bronchus.

Answer 4

There are reticular (linear) and nodular (small round opacities) shadows throughout both lungs, particularly in the middle and the lower zones, obscuring the vessel and heart margins. The reticular shadows form a honeycomb pattern. This is the classic chest radiograph appearance of fibrosing alveolitis.

This case demonstrates the chest radiographic changes of interstitial lung disease as opposed to the air space shadows of acinar or alveolar disease. Although many lung diseases show features of interstitial and air space shadows, a division into the predominant patterns aids the interpreter of the chest radiograph in making a diagnosis.

The characteristic feature of fibrosing alveolitis is the interstitial thickening surrounding cystlike air spaces in a fairly uniform manner, mainly at the periphery of the lungs, as demonstrated on the high resolution CT scan of the thorax (Figure A4).

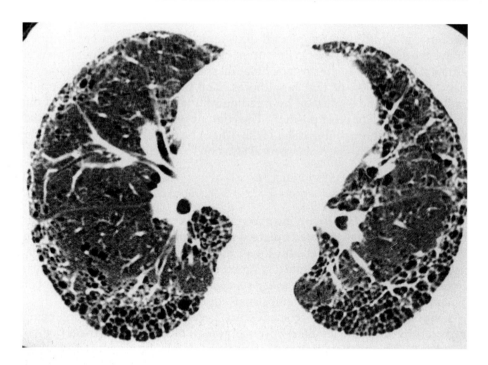

Figure A4

Answer 5

There is an increase in the interstitial shadowing throughout both lungs, as demonstrated by a loss of clarity of the pulmonary vessels and interlobular septal lines (Kerley B lines) in the costopharynx angles (Figure A5). There is upper lobe blood diversion. There is an increase in the reticular pattern in the lower zones and basal pleural effusions. There is an 8 cm calcified left ventricular aneurysm at the apex of the heart which is secondary to a previous myocardial infarction. This is the cause of the Grade 2 pulmonary venous hypertension.

The signs of pulmonary venous hypertension on an erect chest radiograph are graded as follows: Grade 1 (pulmonary artery wedge pressure 14–19 mmHg) is where the diameter of the upper lobe vessel is greater than the lower lobe vessels at a similar distance away from the hilum. The increase in pulmonary venous pressure leads to effacement of the hilar angle and the diameter of the vessels in the first anterior interspace (between the first and second ribs) becomes greater than the normal 3 mm.

Grade 2 (pulmonary artery wedge pressure 20–25 mmHg in acute and 20–30 mmHg in chronic myocardial disease) is characterized by signs of interstitial pulmonary oedema. The fluid causes thickening of the interlobular septa (Kerley B lines). These lines are seen in the most peripheral part of the lungs on the chest radiograph where vessels are normally too small to be seen. Septal lines are 1 mm thick, less than 2 cm in length and are perpendicular to the pleural surface. They are normally located in the lower zones (Figure A5) but can extend up to the mid-zones as in this case. Interstitial space fluid also causes loss of clarity of vessel margins (perihilar haze and perivascular cuffing) and an increase in the reticular pattern in the lower zone. Although interlobular septal lines disappear following treatment of acute pulmonary venous hypertension, they will remain if fibrous thickening of the interlobular septa occurs with chronic raised pulmonary venous hypertension. Other causes of persistent interlobular septal lines on the chest radiograph include pneumoconiosis, lymphangitis carcinomatosis and sarcoidosis.

Grade 3 (pulmonary artery wedge pressure >25 mmHg in acute and >30 mmHg in chronic myocardial disease) pulmonary venous hypertension is characterized by fluid filling the acinar air spaces (consolidation). This causes the 'Batwing' perihilar pattern of consolidation seen in alveolar pulmonary oedema. This may progress to a more extensive distribution. Unilateral alveolar pulmonary oedema can be due to gravity.

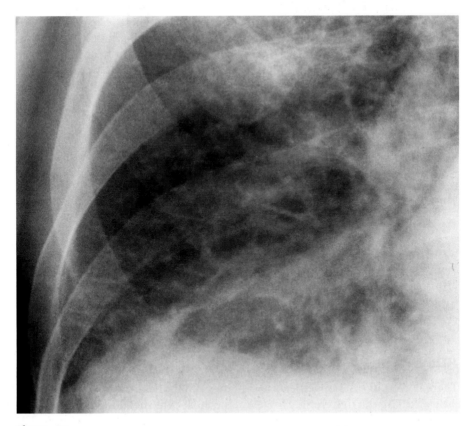

Figure A5

Answer 6

There is bilateral extensive and mainly confluent consolidation throughout both lungs but mainly perihilar in distribution. An air bronchogram is present, being best seen adjacent to the left hilum. In the upper zones, patchy consolidation is due to acinar shadowing (4–10 mm diameter). This is the classic appearance of Grade 3 pulmonary oedema due to pulmonary venous hypertension and indicates that the pulmonary artery wedge pressure is over 25 mmHg. An intraoperative myocardial infarction should be considered and serial cardiac enzymes and electrocardiographs are necessary investigations. A Swan–Ganz catheter should be inserted so that the pulmonary artery wedge pressure and cardiac output can be monitored during inotropic support. The laboratory investigations confirmed that the patient had suffered from an intraoperative myocardial infarction and the pulmonary oedema cleared within 36 hours with appropriate therapy.

Answer 7

The cardiothoracic ratio is 66% (normal is up to 50%). There is an enlarged left atrial appendage (just below the pulmonary artery) and a double right heart border (due to left atrial enlargement). There is thickening of the interlobular septa (Kerley B lines) and a general reticular pattern. In addition, the clarity of the vessel margins is lost and there is upper lobe blood diversion. Nodules of greater soft tissue density are present throughout the lungs. These are the classic chest radiograph signs of mitral stenosis with Grade 2 pulmonary venous hypertension, pulmonary haemosiderosis and ossific nodules. Clearly the cardiac failure requires treatment before a general anaesthetic. In addition, prophylactic antibiotics should be administered before surgical procedures in the mouth, genitourinary tract or gastrointestinal tract to prevent infective endocarditis.

Answer 8

Structure labelled No. 1 is the left cephalic vein. Unopacified blood from the axillary vein causes a streak artefact within the left subclavian vein (structure 2). This joins the left jugular vein to form the left brachiocephalic vein (structure 3). Structure 4 is the right subclavian vein, 5 the right brachiocephalic vein and 6 the superior vena cava.

Answer 9

There is ground glass opacification (a sign of interstitial lung disease), particularly affecting the right lung. However, the most extensive lung pattern is that of consolidation as demonstrated by the air bronchograms in both lungs. The appearances are those of adult respiratory distress syndrome. The pulmonary oedema is due to increased pulmonary vascular permeability, the lung injury in this case being the result of acute smoke inhalation and burns.

The list of causes is extensive, the major groups being sepsis, hypovolaemic shock, trauma, major surgery, burns, bowel infarction, fat embolism, amniotic fluid embolism, aspiration, inhalation injury, metabolic disorders (acute pancreatitis, diabetic ketoacidosis, uraemia), haematological disorders (disseminated intravascular coagulation, leukoaglutinin reactions) and drug-related (heroin, salicylates, methadone).

Answer 10

There is a 5 cm diameter ill-defined cavitating opacity in the left upper zone. A linear tomogram of the apicoposterior segment of the left lung demonstrates the cavity better than the chest radiograph (Figure A10). Patchy foci of

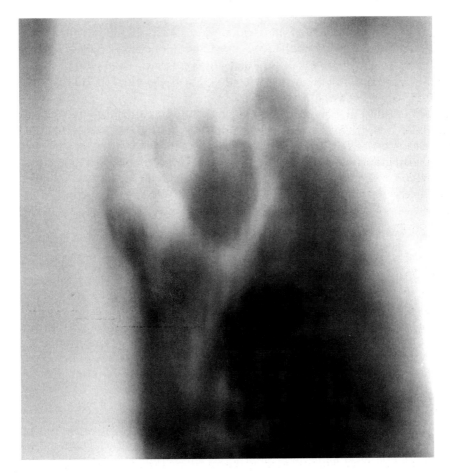

Figure A10

consolidation within the left lower zone and right upper zone are due to bronchopneumonia. These are the appearances of active postprimary *Mycobacterium tuberculosis*.

The initial lesion of postprimary *Mycobacterium tuberculosis* arises in the apicoposterior segment of an upper lobe or the apical segment of a lower lobe in 95% of cases, often with cavitation. Bronchogenic spread leads to bronchopneumonia as in this case. Other causes of cavitating lung lesions include abscesses (*Staphylococcus aureus*, *Klebsiella pneumoniae*, Gram-negative organisms and aspiration pneumonia), neoplasms (squamous cell carcinoma), lung infarction, granulomas, haematomas, cystic bronchiectasis and infected emphysematous bullae. The central, rounded, regular nature of the cavity margin is most often seen in benign lesions. Cavitations in malignant lung masses are typically eccentric and irregular in outline.

Answer 11

Bilateral hilar enlargement and widening of the right side of the superior mediastinum is due to lymphadenopathy. Reticulonodular shadows throughout both lungs indicate interstitial involvement. This patient has the radiological features of sarcoidosis. On clinical examination he had uveitis and erythema nodosa.

The normal hilar shadow on the chest radiograph principally consists of pulmonary arteries and veins. The vessels branch from the normal hilum with no opacities between these diverging branches, apart from the overlying caudally directed main pulmonary arteries. If additional opacities are seen within these diverging branches (as in this case) then a hilar mass should be suspected. In this instance it is due to lymphadenopathy.

Answer 12

There is a right subphrenic hypoechoic collection of fluid in the perihepatic space displacing the liver inferiorly and the right hemidiaphragm superiorly. In the image on the right, the measurement lines demonstrate the size of the fluid collection: 10x35 mm. The collection has some internal echoes within it, consistent with the debris in an abscess. Following diagnostic ultrasound-guided needle aspiration, a percutaneous drainage tube was inserted to drain this subphrenic abscess.

Answer 13

The heart is enlarged (cardiothoracic ratio 0.6). The main pulmonary arterial trunk and the central pulmonary arteries are enlarged. The aortic arch is small. These radiological signs indicate a large left-to-right cardiac shunt due to congenital heart disease. If the patient is undergoing dental, genitourinary tract or gastrointestinal tract surgery then prophylactic antibiotics should be administered to prevent infective endocarditis.

A left-to-right cardiac shunt is the most common congenital heart anomaly. The shunt may be through an atrial septal defect, a ventricular septal defect or an aortopulmonary shunt. If the shunt is large (a shunt ratio of greater than 2:1) as in this case then the main pulmonary arterial trunk and arteries enlarge to compensate for the increase in blood volume. The heart enlarges to reflect the shunt volume overload. The volume of blood delivered to the aorta is reduced so the aortic arch is small (except in cases of patent ductus arteriosus where the shunt is distal to the arch). Echocardiography is required to define the congenital heart defects. There is a risk of endocarditis in cases of atrial septal defects with endocardial cushion defects (as the mitral and tricuspid valves are affected), ventricular septal defects and aortopulmonary shunts. MRI is increasingly being used in demonstrating morphology and function in congenital cardiac disease.

Answer 14

Cystic spaces and linear opacities directed towards the hilum are seen in both lower zones. There is loss of volume of the right lower lobe as demonstrated by the displacement of the right hilum and the horizontal fissure downwards (arrow). There is consolidation, particularly affecting the right lower zone. These are the radiological features of cystic bronchiectasis with infective exacerbation.

The cystic structures demonstrated on the chest radiograph are due to irreversible dilatation of the terminal bronchi. The linear opacities are thickwalled dilated bronchi. Bronchiectasis leads to fibrotic changes with an increase in interstitial shadowing and some loss of volume (the right lower lobe in this case). Infective exacerbation leads to consolidation. Fluid levels sometimes develop in cystic bronchiectasis, particularly during exacerbations of infection.

Answer 15

There is flattening of the left hemidiaphragm and pleural thickening involving the right hemidiaphragm. The right lung is hypertransradient due to large bullae which are demonstrated by hairline walls. The distorted vascular markings extend out to the periphery of the lung. In the left lung there is generalized accentuation of the bronchovascular markings and small, poorly defined opacities indicating interstitial thickening. The right lung demonstrates the bullous changes of emphysema and the left lung demonstrates the 'dirty chest' appearance of chronic bronchitis. However, there are emphysematous changes in the left lung which have caused flattening of the left hemidiaphragm. Thoracic spine scoliosis is noted.

Management: do not put a chest drain in the right hemithorax!

Chronic bronchitis is defined in clinical terms as occurring in patients with expectoration on most days during at least three consecutive months for more than two years. Approximately 50% of such patients have normal chest radiographs. Emphysema is a morphological definition of an increase in size of the air space distal to the terminal bronchioles due either to destruction or dilatation of their walls. Radiologically, this leads to overinflating of the lungs with resultant flattening of the hemidiaphragm. The curvature of the hemidiaphragm is measured by drawing a line from the costophrenic to the cardiophrenic angle and measuring the largest perpendicular to the diaphragm, a value of less than 1.5 cm indicating flattening. The vascular changes of emphysema seen on the chest radiograph include reduction in the size and number of mid-field and peripheral vessels with enlargement of hilar vessels. If the emphysema is predominantly basal then upper lobe blood diversion occurs. In many cases, bullae are most prominent in the upper lobes, in which case there is compression of the lower lobes with crowding of vascular markings at the bases. Bullae are a feature of emphysema; they vary greatly in size and one can be large enough to occupy a hemithorax.

Answer 16

Structure 1 is the endotracheal tube with its tip adequately above the carina. When the head is in neutral position the tip of the endotracheal tube should lie in the mid-trachea, 5–7 cm above the carina. There is an approximate descent of the endotracheal tube of 2 cm when the neck is flexed and an approximate ascent of 3 cm when the neck is extended. Structure 2 is the Swan-Ganz catheter with its tip in the correct position of the pulmonary trunk. Coiled loops within the right atrium or ventricle should be avoided. Structure 3 is a cardiac monitor lead. Structure 4 is the tip of the nasogastric tube seen in the fundus of the stomach.

There are extensive air space shadows throughout both lungs resulting in bilateral air bronchograms. There is blunting of both costophrenic angles due to small bilateral pleural effusions. The cause in this case is due to amniotic fluid embolism leading to adult respiratory distress syndrome.

Answer 17

The patient is rotated to the right. There is a large leftsided pneumothorax, manifested by the visible visceral pleural line and a large radiolucent pleural space devoid of vessels. The immediate management is the insertion of a leftsided chest drain.

The left cardiac border has a clear outline; this is an important sign when trying to identify a small supine pneumothorax. In this case there is an expiratory tension pneumothorax, causing downward displacement of the left hemidiaphragm. The widespread patchy consolidation with an ill-defined nodular, non-segmental pattern, seen in the right lung, occurs in adult respiratory distress syndrome. The tip of the central line is in the right atrium.

Answer 18

There is a sharp radiolucent line crossing the right lambdoid suture; this is due to a fracture involving the right parietal and occipital bones. Linear skull fractures are clearcut, typically straight, cross normal anatomical features such as sutures and do not branch. These features distinguish them from vascular impressions on the skull vault.

If the history of the cause of the fracture sounds implausible then non-accidental injury (child abuse) should be considered as a possible diagnosis. Following a full history and examination, a skeletal survey may be necessary. In non-accidental injury, there are often multiple fractures of varying age.

Answer 19

There is unilateral elevation of the left hemidiaphragm. Loops of bowel are demonstrated below it. The mediastinum is deviated to the right. These are the classic appearances of eventration of the left hemidiaphragm.

A congenital failure in muscular development leads to eventration of the hemidiaphragm. Large eventrations usually affect the left hemidiaphragm. Small localized eventrations or diaphragmatic humps are often seen. It may be difficult to differentiate between diaphragmatic rupture and eventration in a patient with a history of abdominal trauma or upper abdominal surgery. Reference to previous chest radiographs may give the answer. However, if there are none available then in order to diagnose diaphragmatic rupture it is necessary to demonstrate viscera herniating through a diaphragmatic defect and barium studies may be necessary.

Answer 20

Multiple pulmonary nodules are demonstrated throughout both lungs. They are of varying sizes, from 3 mm to 3.5 cm diameter. The nodules are of soft tissue density with smooth margins. No calcification or cavitation is identified within them. The most likely diagnosis is that of multiple pulmonary metastases from a thyroid or renal carcinoma, testicular tumour, sarcoma or lymphoma. In this case the lung metastases were secondary to an asymptomatic seminoma.

The large variation in size of the nodules is characteristic of metastatic deposits. Differential diagnosis to be considered are abscesses, coccidioidomycosis, histoplasmosis, hydatid, Wegener's granulomatosis, rheumatoid nodules, Caplan's syndrome, progressive massive fibrosis and arteriovenous malformations.

Answer 21

There are large (up to 8.5 cm in diameter) smooth-margined lobulated nodules in both mid-zones. Small specks of irregular calcification are seen within them. There is reticulonodular shadowing throughout both lungs and thickened septal lines (Kerley B lines) above the right costophrenic angle. The diagnosis is coalworkers' pneumoconiosis with progressive massive fibrosis (the mid-zone nodules).

The large bilateral nodules with small specks of calcification on background lung changes of pneumoconiosis leave little doubt about the diagnosis of progressive massive fibrosis. In time, the nodules will gradually retract medially, with emphysema developing on their lateral aspects. The nodules sometimes undergo cavitation, in which case superadded tuberculosis has to be excluded.

Answer 22

An 11 cm diameter rounded opacity containing air is seen behind the cardiac shadow. This is a large sliding hiatus hernia. The complications include gastro-oesophageal reflux, aspiration pneumonia and incarceration.

The lateral chest radiograph (Figure A22) demonstrates the hiatus hernia as a posterior mediastinal mass (arrows). Upward herniation of the stomach through the oesophageal hiatus is a common finding. The herniation of abdominal contents through the diaphragm into the thorax can occur as a result of traumatic diaphragmatic tears and congenital defects. The Bochdalek defect is posterolateral through the pleuroperitoneal canal and can present at birth with respiratory distress; 90% are leftsided. The Morgagni hernia is usually an asymptomatic incidental finding, appearing as an anterior soft tissue opacity or air-containing viscus in the right cardiophrenic angle.

Answer 23

Arrow number 1 is indicating an air–fluid level within the sphenoid sinus. No. 2 – the anterior arch of the atlas. No. 3 – the odontoid process of the axis. No. 4 – the top of the vertebral body of T1 which must be seen on all lateral views of the cervical spine following trauma. No. 5 – the retropharyngeal soft tissue anterior to C3. No. 6 – the hard palate. No. 7 – the soft palate. No. 8 – the body of the hyoid. No. 9 – the epiglottis. No. 10 – the vestibule of the larynx.

Apart from the air–fluid level with the sphenoid sinus suggesting a fracture of the base of the skull or sinusitis, the lateral cervical spine view is normal. In the short term, the suspected base of the skull fracture will require antibiotics to prevent meningitis. In assessing the cervical spine following trauma, the interpreter reviews the soft tissues to look for signs of haematoma. With a 2m target/film distance, the thickness of the soft tissues anterior to the body of C3

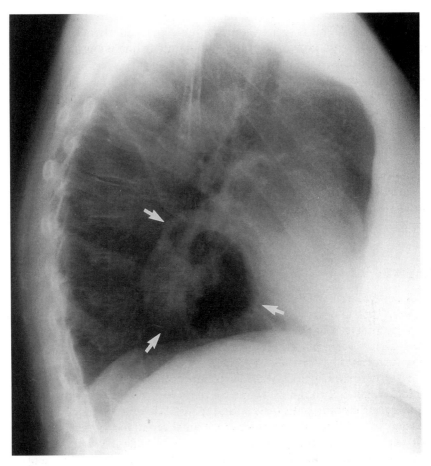

Figure A22

does not normally exceed 7 mm in adults or children prior to endotracheal intubation. False positive measurements can occur due to flexion, expiration and lymphoid tissue hyperplasia, particularly in children. The interpreter checks for fractures and normal alignment. The normal distance between the posterior surface of the anterior arch of the atlas and the anterior surface of the odontoid process is up to 3 mm in adults and up to 5 mm in children. Normal cervical spine alignment is checked for by five lines (Figure A23); 1. the anterior spinal line, which indicates the position of the anterior longitudinal ligament; 2. the posterior spinal line which indicates the position of the posterior longitudinal ligament; 3. line drawn along the posterior cortex of the articular masses; 4. the spinolaminar line drawn at the posterior aspect of the spinal canal; and 5. the spinous process line drawn through the tips of the spinous processes. There is a natural lordosis of the cervical spine. Loss of this lordosis may be due to posture or muscle spasm. Anterior and posterior spinal lines can be disrupted by the normal physiological subluxation of the upper vertebral bodies. This is seen in some patients, particularly in children, due to ligamentous laxity. However, if the spinolaminar line is normal then physiological subluxation is the likely cause.

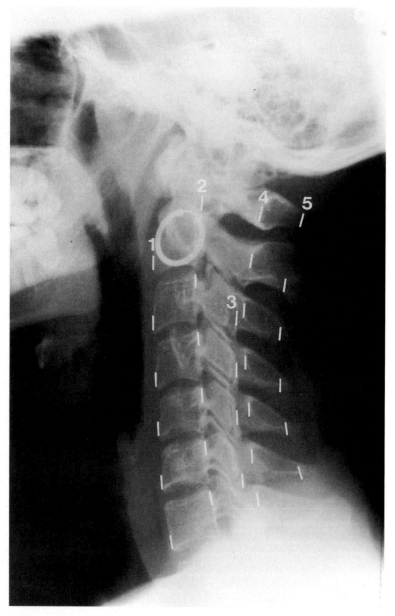

Figure A23

Answer 24

The horizontal fissure has moved upwards. Some air is still present within the right upper lobe, so that it is not completely opaque. The right lower lobe is more transradient than the left lung. This is a case of right upper lobe collapse. The patient requires chest physiotherapy. If this does not result in re-expansion of the right upper lobe then bronchoscopic removal of the mucus plug is required.

Right upper lobe collapse causes the horizontal fissure to move upwards, rotating about the hilum. The right upper lobe lies adjacent to the trachea and superior vena cava, as demonstrated in Figure Q24. The right mediastinal border is effaced (i.e. the silhouette sign). The right lower lobe is more transradient than the contralateral lung because compensatory hyperinflation results in spreading of the lower lobe vessels.

On the lateral projection (Figure A24) the horizontal and oblique fissures are displaced superiorly and anteriorly respectively (arrows). The right upper lobe opacity may be lost in the overlapping shoulder girdle and arm opacities.

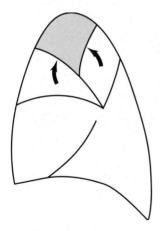

Figure A24

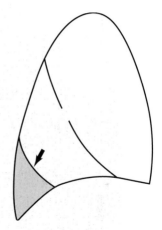

Figure A25

Answer 25

There is flattening of the right hemidiaphragm indicating air trapping due to emphysema. The trachea is deviated to the left and there is loss of volume of the left hemithorax. The left lung appears hypertransradient in comparison to the right due to wider spacing of the vessels. There is a triangular opacity behind the heart arising from the left hilum and descending to the left hemidiaphragm. In conclusion, this is a patient with the lung changes of emphysema who has a left lower lobe collapse which is most likely to be due to a central primary bronchogenic carcinoma. Endoscopy is advised.

The left and right lower lobes collapse posteriorly, caudally and medially as demonstrated by the illustration of a lateral chest radiograph (Figure A25); the oblique fissure is displaced posteriorly and caudally (arrow). In this case there is complete aeration of the left lower lobe and the effacement of the middle and posterior mediastinum becomes an important feature.

Answer 26

There is increased shadowing in the region of the right middle lobe (identified by the loss of the normal right cardiac border, i.e. silhouette sign). Elevation of

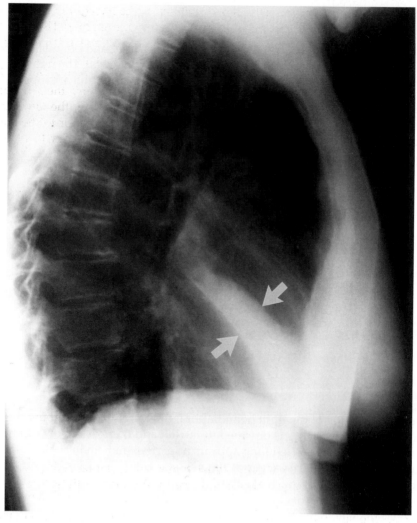

Figure A26

the right hemidiaphragm indicates some volume loss. The right horizontal (minor) fissure is displaced downwards, pivoting about the hilum. These are the signs of a right middle lobe collapse (arrows), best demonstrated on the right lateral radiograph (Figure A26). There is a rounded right hilar mass, which is a bronchogenic carcinoma causing the right middle lobe collapse.

Answer 27

There are patchy areas of consolidation within the right lung, becoming confluent in the right lower lobe. There is a veil-like opacification of the left lung with sparing of the left lower lobe. Effacement of the left tracheal margin and left heart border is noted (silhouette sign). Deviation of the trachea to the left and a raised left hemidiaphragm indicate loss of volume of the left lung. These are the features of aspiration pneumonia and left upper lobe collapse. If the left upper lobe does not respond to physiotherapy then endoscopy may be required.

The oblique fissure (arrows) moves anteriorly during collapse of the left upper lobe (Figure A27). This is because the lingula prevents the left upper lobe being a mirror image collapse of the right upper lobe. If the lower lobe hyperinflates sufficiently, the collapsed upper lobe lies anterior to the aortic knuckle, which then becomes visible. The radiolucency anterior to the collapsed left upper lobe is due to herniation of the right lung.

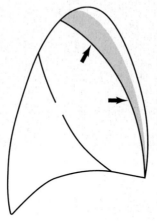

Figure A27

Answer 28

There is a large retrosternal goitre causing marked deviation of the trachea to the right. Prior knowledge of this is important as the anaesthetist can anticipate a difficult intubation.

The coronal T1 weighted magnetic resonance image (Figure A28) demonstrates the intrathoracic extent of the goitre. The goitre, which contains

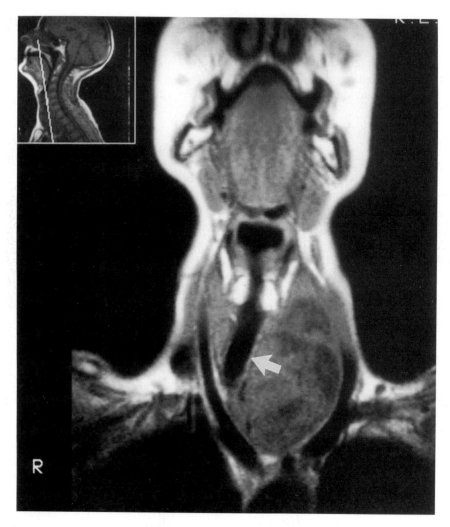

Figure A28

inhomogeneous signal, extends down to the aortic arch and is displacing the trachea to the right (arrow).

Other causes of anterior mediastinal masses which may displace and narrow the trachea are enlarged lymph nodes in lymphoma, and thymoma. The superior mediastinal mass in this case obviously extends up into the neck, making a retrosternal goitre the most likely diagnosis.

Answer 29

There is surgical emphysema in the left thoracic wall, left axilla and left arm. This means that there is a puncture of the parietal pleural, with the likelihood

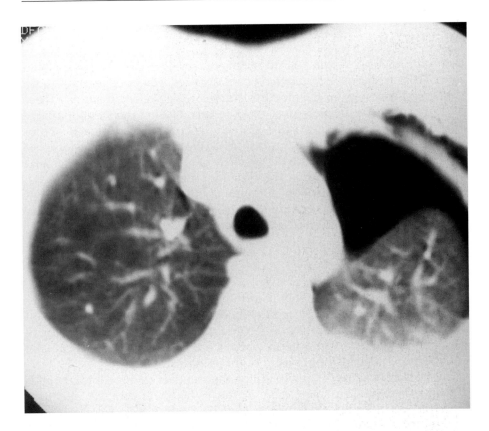

Figure A29

of a visceral pleural rupture and a pneumothorax. The signs demonstrated in this case are: the left mediastinal border is seen with more clarity than normal, consistent with a pneumothorax; fractures of the outer end of the left clavicle and the posterior part of the second left rib are noted. An erect or lateral decubitus chest radiograph would confirm the diagnosis.

The CT scan of the thorax taken 30 minutes after the chest radiograph demonstrates the anterior position of air in a supine pneumothorax. Air in the pleural space in a supine patient collects in the highest region which is the anterior costophrenic sulcus. On a supine chest radiograph this will produce a radiolucency of the upper abdominal quadrant, lower thorax and the costophrenic angle. The diaphragm may be displaced downwards. Pleural air tends to lie in a subpulmonary region and may outline the visceral pleural line of the lung base. As more air enters the pleural space the cardiac outline is seen with greater clarity.

Answer 30

There are ill-defined nodules of consolidation, varying in size, throughout both lungs. These are the classic radiographic appearances of fat embolism syndrome.

Fat droplets can enter the bloodstream following skeletal fractures. These 20–40 mm diameter droplets cause small vessel occlusion and vasculitis in the lungs, brain, kidneys and skin. The fat embolism syndrome develops 12–48 hours following skeletal trauma. This is the time it takes for tissue lipase to hydrolyse the neutral fat droplets to form free fatty acids that have the toxic effect on vascular endothelium. The ill-defined nodular air space shadows can develop into more confluent opacification of the lungs. Clearing of the lungs takes between seven and 14 days unless the complication of adult respiratory distress syndrome supervenes, as in this case.

Answer 31

The cardiothoracic ratio is enlarged, there is a bulging of the left cardiac border and enlargement of the main pulmonary artery. There is effacement of the normal right cardiac silhouette, suggesting that there is an abnormality of the right middle lobe. The anterior ends of the ribs are sloping abnormally downwards. These are the appearances of pectus excavatum.

The chest radiograph of this condition can simulate cardiac and right middle lobe disease. The shadowing in the right lower zone is due to a combination of the normal soft tissues of the chest wall, as they funnel obliquely inwards, and vascular markings which are conspicuous now that the heart is deviated to the left. Clinically, an examination of the patient confirms the diagnosis. Preoperative assessment necessitates a lateral radiograph (Figure A31). The posterior border of the sternum is arrowed.

Answer 32

On the anteroposterior view the normal line of the spinous processes is disrupted with the spinous process of C4 deviated to the left. On the lateral radiograph there is mild anterior subluxation of C4 on C5 with disruption of all the five spinal lines. The posterior surface of the articular masses of C4 and C3 are not superimposed, indicating a rotational deformity at the C4 level. There is a fracture of the left articular mass of C5. There is a small avulsion fracture of the anterosuperior surface of the body of C5, indicating disruption of the anterior longitudinal ligament. The diagnosis is a unilateral facet dislocation of the left C4/C5 facet, caused by a hyperflexion and rotation injury. Unilateral facet dislocation injuries are usually initially stable. However, in this case there has been disruption of the anterior longitudinal ligament and fracture of the left articular mass of C5. This is an unstable injury, necessitating reduction and fixation.

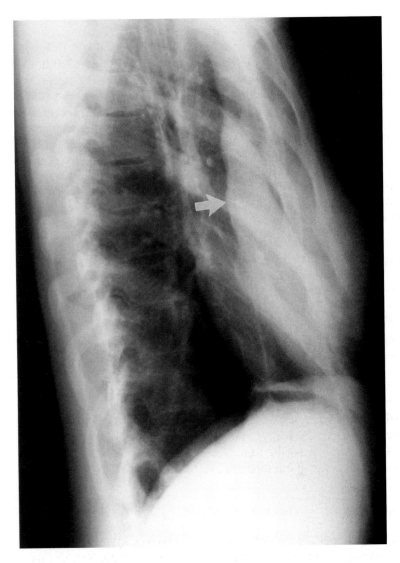

Figure A31

When is a spinal injury stable or unstable? This depends upon the extent of bone and ligamentous injury involved. Fractures can be assessed with plain radiographs and CT. However, disruption of the ligamentum flavum, the anterior and posterior longitudinal ligaments, the interspinous, supraspinous and intertransverse ligaments, as well as the joint capsule, is diagnosed by recognizing the features of subluxation and avulsion fractures. As a guideline, cervical instability has been described when there is more than 3.5 mm horizontal displacement of a vertebra or more than 11° of hyperflexion. Unfortunately, cervical radiography may appear normal in the presence of an unstable cervical spine injury following some hyperextension injuries. The subtle signs of an unstable injury include prevertebral soft tissue swelling, widening of the intervertebral disc space and the interfacet joints and splaying of the spinous processes. Magnetic resonance imaging is able to demonstrate the extent of acute spinal cord injury and has the advantage of being able to demonstrate ligamentous injury, herniated intervertebral discs and haematomas. Flexion and extension views can also be performed within an MR scanner in order to show functional subluxation. The disadvantage of MRI is that it does not demonstrate bone fragments as well as plain radiography or CT.

Answer 33

The heart is deviated to the right and the left cardiac border is seen with more clarity than usual. The upper left abdominal quadrant, lower left thorax and left costophrenic angles are more radiolucent than normal. This is the appearance of a leftsided pneumothorax on a supine radiograph. A decubitus film

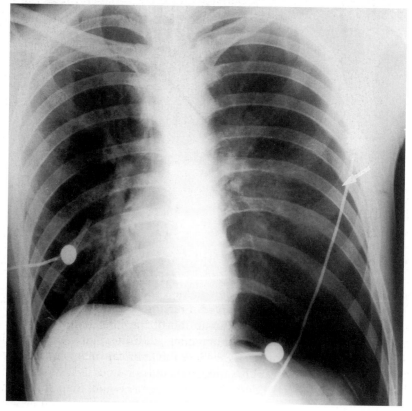

Figure A33

with the left side raised or an erect chest radiograph will confirm this prior to inserting a chest drain.

The patient's condition deteriorated and another supine radiograph taken 30 minutes later (Figure A33) demonstrated a visible visceral pleural line (arrow).

Answer 34

There is free peritoneal air, which is well demonstrated by air tracking into the perihepatic space between the superior surface of the liver and inferior surface of the right hemidiaphragm. In this clinical context the free peritoneal air is most likely to be due to a perforated peptic ulcer. Other causes of perforated viscus to consider are diverticular disease, bowel infarction, gastrointestinal malignancy and intestinal obstruction.

The radiographic technique is important to identify small amounts of free peritoneal gas. Either a well-penetrated erect chest radiograph or, if the patient

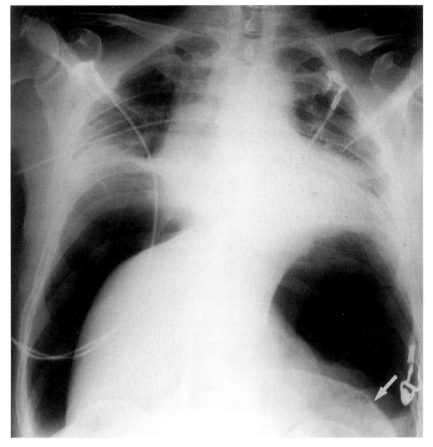

Figure A34

cannot stand or sit up, a right lateral decubitus abdominal radiograph is taken. The patient remains in that position for ten minutes before the radiograph is taken, to allow the free gas to rise within the abdomen. The erect chest radiograph of another patient (Figure A34), with a massive pneumoperitoneum from perforated large bowel, demonstrates air on both sides of the bowel wall (arrow). This is an important radiological sign of free peritoneal air on supine abdominal radiographs. In this case there is bilateral lower lobe atelectasis.

Answer 35

There is an air-containing viscus in the right cardiophrenic angle. This is a Morgagni hernia with incarceration of the antrum and pyloris of the stomach causing gastric outlet obstruction. A previous thoracoplasty of the left upper lobe and emphysematous bullae in the left lower lobe are noted.

Barium meal examination demonstrates the herniation of the stomach body and antrum through the anterior diaphragmatic defect (arrow) in the lateral projection.

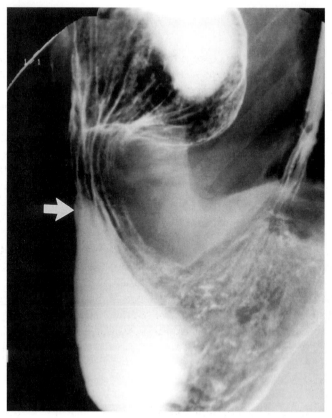

Figure A35

Answer 36

The visceral pleural line of the collapsed right lung is identifiable, indicating a large rightsided pneumothorax. The mediastinum is deviated to the left and there is herniation of pleural air to the left. There are small nodular opacities throughout the lung and the vascular structures are obscured, indicating interstitial lung disease. This patient is suffering from a pneumothorax secondary to her *Pneumocystis carinii* pneumonia. A chest drain relieved her acute symptoms.

Patients with early *Pneumocystis carinii* pneumonia may show no abnormality on the chest radiograph. In such cases the threshold of radiographic visibility has not been reached even though gallium 67 lung scans are positive. The earliest radiographic signs are of a diffuse small nodular pattern (as in this case) of interstitial lung disease with some sparing of the peripheral lung and apices. As the disease progresses, diffuse consolidation develops. A spontaneous pneumothorax is a recognized complication of *Pneumocystis carinii* pneumonia and usually follows rupture of a pneumatocele, which is localized peripheral focus air trapping. Pneumatoceles are identifiable on a chest radiograph prior to their rupture.

Answer 37

A 4 cm diameter smooth-margined mass lies adjacent to the lower part of the right hilum. It has a homogeneous density with no calcification or cavitation. This mass is due to a primary bronchogenic carcinoma. In addition, there is a holly leaf-shaped, inhomogeneous opacity adjacent to the upper part of the right hilum. This is a pleural plaque.

Inhalation of asbestos fibres can cause pleural plaques (as in this case), calcified pleural plaques, pleural effusion and mesotheliomas. The lung parenchyma can be affected by asbestosis (not seen in this case) leading to an increase in the interstitial shadows in the mid-zones and bases. Carcinoma of the bronchus is more common in patients with asbestosis. It is debatable whether or not there is an increased incidence of carcinoma of the bronchus associated with pleural plaques.

Calcified pleural plaques mainly occur in the parietal pleura over the lower zones, the heart and diaphragm. Look for fibrous pleural plaques at the lung periphery – just under the lateral portions of the ribs is a characteristic site. CT is helpful not only in establishing the presence of pleural plaques, but also in demonstrating pulmonary fibrosis due to asbestos exposure.

Pleural effusion, which may rapidly diminish or increase in size, is a less common feature of asbestos exposure.

Answer 38

The inco-ordination of this patient's swallowing has lead to barium entering the trachea as well as the oesophagus. A small, rounded pharyngeal pouch is seen in association with the impaired relaxation of the cricopharyngeus. This patient's right basal consolidation was attributed to chronic aspiration pneumonia. She will require chest physiotherapy to help remove the barium from the right lower lobe.

Answer 39

Structure 1 is a convex–concave acute on chronic subdural haematoma.
Structure 2 is the frontal sinus of the frontal bone.
Structure 3 is the left frontal lobe.
Structure 4 is the frontal horn of the left lateral ventricle.
Structure 5 is the sylvian fissure.
Structure 6 is the normal calcified choroid plexus within the left lateral ventricle.
Structure 7 is the left occipital lobe.
Structure 8 is the falx cerebri.

The diagnosis is an acute on chronic subdural haematoma causing herniation of the brain to the left and compression of the right lateral ventricle.

Subdural haematomas occur when a deceleration injury causes the bridging veins between the cerebral cortex and the dural sinus to tear, but they sometimes occur spontaneously. The haematoma collects in the space between the inner layer of the dura and the arachnoid membrane. In the acute stage the subdural haematoma appears homogeneously hyperdense (whiter) compared to the cerebral cortex. At approximately 2–3 weeks, the subdural haematoma will become isodense with the cerebral cortex, sometimes making it difficult to detect a small subdural collection. Opacification of the vessels in the subarachnoid space with intravenous contrast medium aids visualization of the subdural haematoma border. Chronic subdural haematomas are homogeneously hypodense (darker) in relation to the cerebral cortex. Acute bleeding within a chronic subdural haematoma is demonstrated as a mixed density, as in this case.

Answer 40

The lungs are overinflated and a symmetrical increase in the reticular (linear) shadows spreads outwards from the hila. There are small bilateral pleural effusions. These are the appearances of transient tachypnoea of the newborn. These babies usually become asymptomatic by 48 hours of age. In this case, a subsequent radiograph (Figure A40) is normal. The wide mediastinal outline is due to the normal thymus (arrows).

Transient tachypnoea of the newborn is the result of delayed resorption of fetal lung fluid, with the resultant radiographic appearances of interstitial pulmonary oedema.

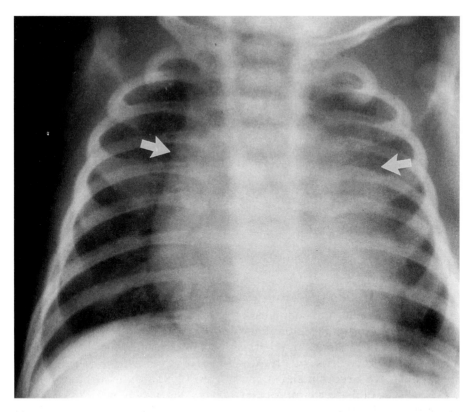

Figure A40

Answer 41

The patient is intubated. There is consolidation involving the right upper and lower lobes. An air bronchogram is demonstrated affecting the right lower lobe. A diagnosis to be considered is ventilator-associated pneumonia (the major pathogens are aerobic Gram-negative bacilli and *Staphylococcus aureus*). The adverse risk factors include duration of mechanical ventilation, aspiration of gastric contents, chronic obstructive airways disease, reintubation, 24-hour mechanical ventilator circuit changes, use of positive end-expiratory pressure, age, multiple organ system failure, prior antibiotic administration, thoracic/upper abdominal surgery, depressed consciousness, supine head position, and histamine type 2 receptor antagonists. The consolidation in this case may be the sterile lung changes of acute inhalation injury. However, the air bronchogram is the most specific radiological sign of ventilator-associated pneumonia. Therefore in the appropriate clinical setting bronchoscopic sampling of the lower airways using a protected specimen brush should be performed, as this is the most accurate method of diagnosing ventilator-associated pneumonia short of direct tissue examination.

Answer 42

The vertebral bodies of C6 and C7 have not been imaged and further radiographs should be obtained. There is prevertebral soft tissue swelling. The five radiological lines of the cervical spine are disrupted at the atlantoaxial level. There is splaying between the spinous processes of the axis and atlas. The odontoid process is fractured at its base and anteriorly displaced. This is an unstable fracture.

The child requires an immobilizing collar, followed by reduction and fixation of the fracture.

Answer 43

In addition to the posterior fractures of the seventh to tenth left ribs, there are fractures of the lateral parts of the fifth to eighth left ribs. There is no evidence of a pneumothorax or lung contusion. There is crowding of the posterior part of the left ribs in the mid and lower zones, indicating poor lung expansion in this region. Some of the ribs have two fractures and there is therefore a flail segment. Analgesia from an intercostal nerve block is required, followed by careful monitoring of her respiratory function.

The classic treatment would be to perform intercostal blocks at the angle of the ribs. A continuous intercostal extrapleural or intercostal intrapleural nerve block could also be considered.

Answer 44

There is a ground glass opacification of both lungs with small nodular elements. The pulmonary vasculature is obscured and the air bronchograms are more prominent than normal. The visceral pleural line of both lungs is identified approximately 3 mm from the ribs. There is a region of confluent consolidation in the apex of the left upper lobe and in the right lower lobe. The diagnosis is hyaline membrane disease with bilateral pneumothoraces and superadded confluent consolidation. This baby is likely to require ventilatory support. If the blood gases do not improve sufficiently then chest drains would need to be inserted. Cultures should be taken from the tracheal aspirate and antibiotics considered. However, the regions of consolidation may be due to pulmonary haemorrhage rather than infection, which tends to clear within 24 hours.

Respiratory distress of the newborn may be due to ventilatory (hyaline membrane disease, aspiration, pneumonia), mechanical (pneumothorax, diaphragmatic hernia, congenital lobular emphysema, cystic adenomatoid malformation) or circulatory (congenital heart disease) causes. The initial radiograph is valuable in diagnosing the particular cause. In some premature babies the Type II alveolar cells are unable to release or produce alveolar surfactant and this leads to collapse of the alveoli. Pulmonary capillaries leak proteins which form hyaline membrane. Patent terminal airways are

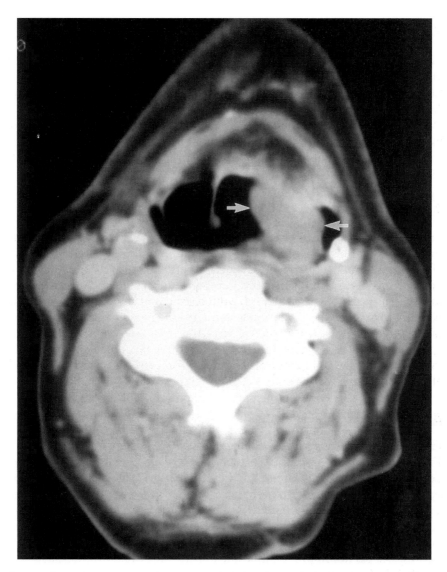

Figure A45

surrounded by fluid-filled alveoli giving a characteristic appearance of small nodules on the chest radiograph. As more alveoli become fluid-filled, the air bronchograms become more prominent.

Answer 45

The lateral soft tissue radiograph of the neck shows a large irregular soft tissue density mass in the region of the epiglottis with posterior displacement of the vestibule. One of the aryepiglottic folds appears lax, while the other is invaded with tumour and appears as a soft tissue density mass in the vestibule. This is due to carcinoma of the larynx affecting the epiglottis and left aryepiglottic fold (arrows), as demonstrated on the contrast enhanced CT (Figure A45).

This patient would present a challenge for endotracheal intubation as visualization of the glottis would require the use of a fibreoptic laryngoscope or bronchoscope. The tumour is too extensive for a shared airway procedure. This tumour is being treated with radiotherapy. However, if laryngectomy was performed a tracheostomy would be necessary.

Answer 46

There is a region of consolidation above the left costophrenic angle; it is hump shaped and is subpleural in location. There is linear atelectasis above the consolidation. Loss of the normal left hemidiaphragm/lung interface (silhouette sign) is due to a leftsided pleural effusion. The combination of hump-shaped subpleural consolidation, linear atelectasis and a pleural effusion are the classic chest radiographic appearances of a pulmonary embolism with lung infarction. Upper lobe blood diversion is noted, indicating Grade I pulmonary venous hypertension.

Management: this patient requires anticoagulation, a confirmatory radio-isotope ventilation and perfusion scan and, if there is still doubt about the diagnosis, a pulmonary angiogram.

Non-specific chest radiograph changes of pulmonary embolism are seen in approximately 50% of cases. The vascular changes include focal vasoconstriction distal to an embolism with resultant regional decrease in the vascular shadows. The artery proximal to an embolism will become dilated. The lung changes include localized regions of collapse (atelectasis), seen as linear or triangular opacities. In addition, unilateral elevation of the hemidiaphragm is often seen. Lung infarction results in a hump-shaped subpleural region of consolidation. A small pleural effusion usually accompanies the pulmonary infarction. A radionuclide lung scan is used to confirm the suspected diagnosis of pulmonary embolism. The radionuclide and pharmaceutical agents used for the perfusion and ventilation studies vary according to the institution. The perfusion scan is a very sensitive but non-specific test for detecting the abnormal distribution of pulmonary artery blood flow and a negative scan effectively rules out pulmonary embolism. The ventilation scan is sensitive in detecting the lung changes of chronic disease (e.g. bullae). A high probability (>95% chance that the diagnosis is pulmonary embolism) ventilation/perfusion scan is one that has >1.5 lung segments with perfusion defects but not ventilation defects, i.e. air still enters these lung segments but they are not perfused. In this case a 99^m technetium labelled microspheres aggregated albumen perfusion scan (Figure A46) demonstrates perfusion defects in the left mid and lower zones and the right lower zone, indicating a high probability of pulmonary embolism. A pulmonary angiogram is the 'gold standard' test. It is

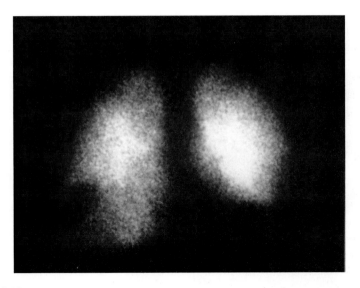

Figure A46

indicated when there is an indeterminate isotope lung scan, prior to embolec-tomy, the insertion of an inferior vena caval filter and use of thrombolytic agents.

Answer 47

Sternotomy wires are noted. There is a smooth-margined mass, approxi-mately 15 cm in diameter and containing punctate calcification, in the left lower lobe behind the heart (the left heart border is clearly seen indicating that the mass is in the posterior part of the thorax). The next step is to review the patient's previous imaging as this lesion is unlikely to be an acute complica-tion of the operation or anaesthesia.

This case demonstrates the important principle of having the previous imaging of a patient available. The CT scan of the thorax (Figure A47) demon-strates the smooth-margined mass and punctate central calcification characteristic of a large hamartoma (arrow). This patient required a coronary artery bypass graft operation and removal of the hamartoma. The former operation was performed first in order to reduce the operative risk for the later operation.

Only 20–30% of hamartomas actually contain calcification. Some hamartomas grow over a period of time, as in this case, thus mimicking a malignant lesion.

Answer 48

A ventriculoperitoneal shunt and a gastrostomy feeding tube are noted. There is a severe >65° scoliosis concave to the left. The left femoral head is dislocated

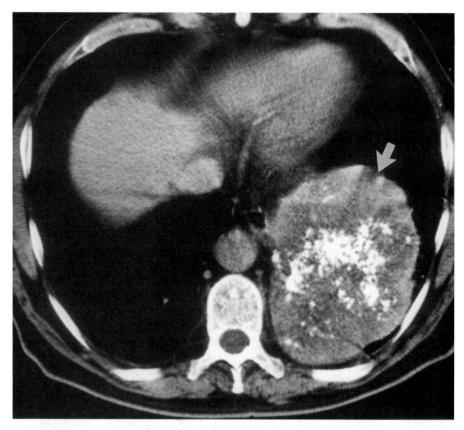

Figure A47

and there is spina bifida from T12 to L3. The severe scoliosis will cause functional changes within the respiratory system. The lateral rotation of the vertebral bodies leads to a concave hypoinflated hemithorax compressed towards residual volume (right hemithorax in this case) and a convex hyperinflated hemithorax expanded towards the total lung capacity of that lung (left hemithorax in this case). The overall decrease in the total lung capacity and the residual volume, and the mechanical impairment lead to alveolar hypoventilation. The ventilation/perfusion mismatch results in a decrease in the arterial oxygen tension and an increase in the arterial carbon dioxide tension. The chronic hypercapniac kyphoscoliotic patient will respond subnormally to further elevations of carbon dioxide tension, and hypoventilates when inhaling high concentrations of oxygen. The chronic hypoxia can lead to an increase in pulmonary vascular resistance, right ventricular hypertrophy and cor pulmonale. Preoperative respiratory function tests should include an assessment of the total lung capacity, vital capacity, residual volume and compliance, in addition to arterial blood gas analysis. An electrocardiogram is necessary to detect cor pulmonale. Patients undergoing spinal fusion for scoliosis will benefit from a deliberate hypotensive technique to reduce blood loss. In these cases postoperative intensive care therapy may be necessary, as respiratory deterioration in the immediate postoperative period is common.

Answer 49

There is an extensive haematoma in the parapharyngeal region causing marked compression of the pharyngeal air space. Air is present in the masseter muscles. A normal coronal CT scan at a similar level is provided for comparison (Figure A49). Clearly in a case of major facial trauma, as in this case, the airway may need to be protected by endotracheal intubation. If this is difficult or there are additional airway problems such as a fractured larynx, then a tracheostomy may be necessary.

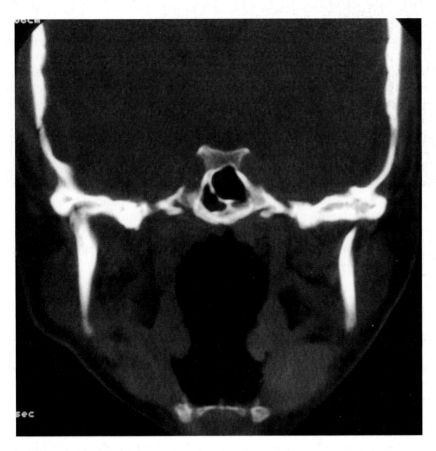

Figure A49

Answer 50

A nasogastric tube lies in the trachea. It is kinked in the right main bronchus and its tip lies in the left lower lobe bronchus. This case illustrates the value of a check chest radiograph when there has been a difficult insertion of a nasogastric tube or when no gastric aspirate is obtained. The same principle also applies to other intubation procedures.

Answer 51

There is air within the fascial planes in the soft tissues of the neck. In addition, a thin line of air outlines the mediastinum. The elevated parietal pleural line is well demonstrated adjacent to the cardiac shadow. The signs indicate a pneumomediastinum. There is consolidation in the right middle lobe, which is most probably due to infection.

The presence of a pneumomediastinum indicates perforation of the respiratory or gastrointestinal tracts. The main causes include (a) alveolar rupture (spontaneous, ventilated patients and trauma) where air tracks through the interstitial tissues; (b) traumatic rupture of the trachea or bronchus; (c) perforation of the oesophagus (spontaneous and postinstrumentation); (d) perforation of the pharynx, duodenum, colon, and rectum with air tracking to the mediastinum; (e) mediastinitis. In comparison, the air of a pneumothorax needs to be demonstrated extending over the apex or lateral border of the lung. Pneumomediastinum following a tracheostomy rarely affects patient outcome. To prevent a tension pneumomediastinum compressing the heart and major vessels, the ventilatory pressure should be reduced to a minimum. If inadvertent placement of the tracheostomy tube into the paratracheal soft tissue or through the posterior tracheal membrane is suspected, a lateral cervical radiograph will demonstrate the anteroposterior relationship of the tip of the tracheostomy tube.

Answer 52

This expiration chest radiograph demonstrates mediastinal shift to the left, due to either collapse of some of the left lung or obstructive air trapping in the right lung pushing the mediastinum over to the left. The chest radiograph taken on arrested inspiration was normal. The child therefore has a foreign body lodged in the right main bronchus.

A chest radiograph taken soon after the aspiration of a foreign body (often a peanut) often demonstrates obstructive overinflation of the affected lobe or lung. Fluoroscopic examination is useful if there is difficulty in obtaining the expiratory film. As the air distal to the obstruction becomes absorbed, then collapse and pneumonia of the affected lobe or lung will be demonstrated on the chest radiograph.

Answer 53

There are two catheters in the venous system. The one on the right lies in the right subclavian vein and its tip is in the superior vena cava. The catheter on the left lies within the left subclavian vein. There is no contrast delineation of the left brachiocephalic vein and superior vena cava. Contrast medium is reaching the right atrium via the left superior intercostal, superior hemiazygos and azygos veins.

The appearances are those of thrombosis within the brachiocephalic veins and superior vena cava leading to the superior vena caval syndrome. The cause in this case is the right central venous catheter. The commonest cause is due to a mediastinal neoplasm (usually carcinoma of the bronchus) but other causes include lymphoma, mediastinal fibrosis and aortic aneurysm. Stenting of the superior vena cava can relieve the distressing symptoms.

Answer 54

There is massive mediastinal widening due to a large mediastinal haematoma. Instrumental injury to the mediastinal veins or arteries has occurred. A dynamic, contrast-enhanced CT scan may be helpful in delineating the bleeding point. If this is negative, then in the case of a particularly large or rapidly expanding mediastinal haemorrhage, an arch aortogram should be considered as there may possibly be damage to the brachiocephalic common carotid or subclavian artery. If this is negative, venogram studies may be necessary.

During the introduction of long lines it is not unusual for iatrogenic mediastinal haematomas to occur. Venous haemorrhage is most often the cause and it is usually self-limiting.

Answer 55

There is a fracture of the body of the sternum. The superior fracture fragment is displaced 1 cm posteriorly. A fracture of the sternum indicates severe trauma and associated injuries to the aorta and branches, heart, superior vena cava, lungs and pleura should be considered. A good quality chest radiograph is therefore essential in these cases.

Answer 56

There is some consolidation in the right mid and lower zones. In the mid-zone there is an air–fluid level with an interface length of 2.5 cm. The right hemidiaphragm is raised and fluid within the pleural space extends nearly to the lung apex. The air–fluid level in the right mid-zone represents a lung abscess in the right upper lobe, with pneumonia of the right upper and lower lobes, as well as an associated pleural effusion which may be an empyema.

Pulmonary contusion following lung trauma represents blood in the alveoli. It has the appearances of consolidation and usually clears within 10–14 days. Pulmonary lacerations, although originally linear, often take on an elliptical shape and appear cystic. Haemorrhage into these cystic spaces leads to an air–fluid level. The laceration may completely fill with blood to form a haematoma, which usually resolves within four months.

One complication of lung laceration is the development of a lung abscess (as in this case).

Answer 57

There is a large air-containing biconvex epidural haematoma compressing the right frontal lobe and causing it to herniate across to the left. The frontal horns of the lateral ventricles are compressed. There is a low density region and loss of the normal grey/white matter differentiation in the left occipital lobe. The subtle appearances are consistent with cerebral oedema due to contusion of a contrecoup injury in this region. There is a large extracranial haematoma adjacent to the right frontal and parietal bones. The next step in this patient's management is immediate transfer to a neurosurgical centre for evacuation of this epidural haematoma and haemostasis.

The presence of air within the haematoma indicates that this is a compound fracture, probably due to a sinus fracture.

Answer 58

A dual chamber permanent pacemaker, sternotomy wires and surgical clips are noted. The cardiothoracic ratio is enlarged and the heart has a globular appearance, suggesting a postoperative pericardial effusion. The effusion was confirmed with an echocardiogram and was drained via a pericardial catheter (arrow) (Figure A58).

Answer 59

There is a predominantly reticulonodular pattern throughout both lungs, with loss of clarity of the normal vascular margins. The hila are prominent and ill defined. There is bilateral blunting of the costophrenic angles due to pleural effusions; these may be malignant pleural effusions. The cardiothoracic ratio is within normal limits. In this clinical context, the appearances are consistent with lymphangitis carcinomatosa.

Metastatic spread to the pulmonary lymphatic system, resulting in lymphangitis carcinomatosa, is most commonly from breast, bronchus, stomach, colon and prostate primary tumours, as well as lymphoma. The thickening of the interstitial tissue from lymphangitis carcinomatosa can give a radiographic appearance similar to interstitial pulmonary oedema and clearly the

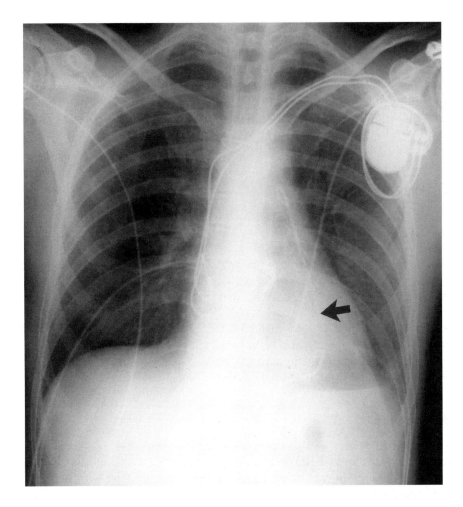

Figure A58

assessment of the cardiothoracic ratio, pulmonary vessels and the clinical information is important to differentiate between the two.

Answer 60

The left lung visceral pleural outline is identified, indicating a large leftsided pneumothorax which requires a chest drain. There is an increase in the linear opacities arising from the hila and extending into the upper lobes, particularly on the left, indicating interstitial pulmonary oedema.

The initial chest radiograph of a patient following near drowning may be entirely normal even though the patient may require ventilatory support. On subsequent films (Figure A60) bilaterally symmetrical consolidation often

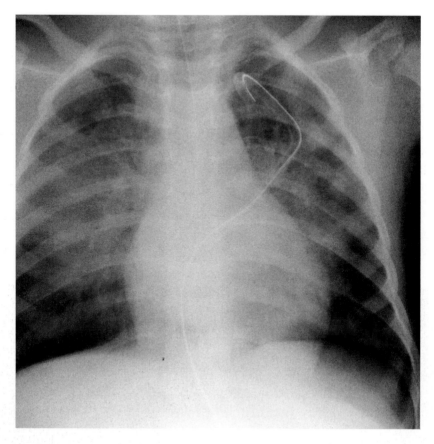

Figure A60

develops. A pneumothorax or pneumomediastinum is a common occurrence in a near drowning victim requiring mechanical ventilation.

Answer 61

There are bilateral patchy areas of consolidation in both lungs. The lungs are overinflated and there is a rightsided pleural effusion. These are the classic appearances of meconium aspiration. Oxygen via a mask may be sufficient to maintain the appropriate blood gas levels. However, endotracheal intubation and ventilation may be required. Careful monitoring for the complications of aspiration and superimposed bacterial infection is necessary.

Aspiration of clear amniotic fluid may occur in babies delivered by caesarean section. These babies usually show a rapid improvement in their respiratory function. Babies born following fetal distress may aspirate meconium-soiled amniotic fluid. They may demonstrate rapid improvement in 24–48 hours or develop the complications described above.

Answer 62

There is curvilinear calcification bordering a soft tissue density mass to the left of the L2–4 vertebral bodies. The mass is greater than 6 cm in transverse diameter. These are the radiographic signs of an aortic aneurysm. There are some coincidental calcified mesenteric lymph nodes to the right of the lumbar spine.

The clinical history suggests that the aneurysm is leaking. If the patient is in shock, an urgent surgical opinion should be sought. Avoid raising the blood pressure above 100 mmHg systolic. If the patient is haemodynamically stable and confirmation of a leaking aneurysm is required, then a dynamically contrast-enhanced CT scan of the abdomen should be performed (Figure A62).

An image from the level of L4 from another patient demonstrates a contrast-enhanced lumen size of 10 cm diameter. Retroperitoneal leakage of blood is demonstrated by the effacement of the left psoas muscle and an

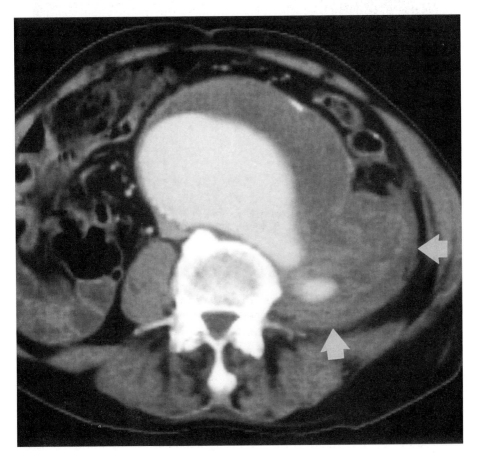

Figure A62

irregular density haematoma in the lower left perinephric space (arrows). On cephalad scans, the aneurysm was shown to lie below the level of the renal arteries.

Answer 63

There is a calcified false aneurysm (pseudoaneurysm) affecting the descending aorta at the level of the ligamentum arteriosum. A left lateral radiograph (Figure A63) shows the pseudoaneurysm (arrow) and the course of the descending aorta (open arrows). On enquiry, this patient gave a history of sternal and rib fractures following a motor vehicle accident some years previously. This false aneurysm should be electively resected.

   The vast majority of patients with aortic rupture due to a rapid deceleration injury die immediately. The shearing forces of fixed points along the aortic wall, particularly at the ligamentum arteriosum, causes traumatic rupture of the aortic wall. In 2–5% of cases, intact aortic adventitia and perivascular connective tissue, together with a haematoma, form a false aneurysm which often eventually calcifies. Delayed rupture and infection can occur at the site of these false aneurysms.

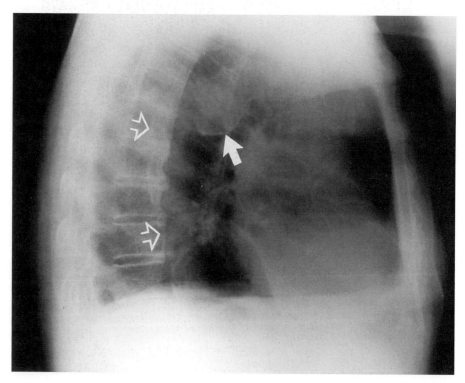

Figure A63

In the acute stage of aortic rupture the clinical picture is of shock, stridor from tracheal compression or superior vena caval syndrome due to hae-matoma. The chest radiograph signs of acute aortic rupture include mediastinal widening, loss of the normal aortic arch contour, endotracheal or nasogastric tube displacement to the right and a depressed left main bron-chus. There may be an associated leftsided haemothorax and fracture of the first to third ribs on the left. With these chest radiographic signs an aortic angiogram is indicated. If the chest radiographic signs are equivocal, CT scan of the mediastinum is required. If a mediastinal bleed is confirmed, then aortography should follow.

Answer 64

The sylvian fissures, the third ventricle and the quadrigeminal plate cistern are filled with a high density fluid which is subarachnoid blood. There is

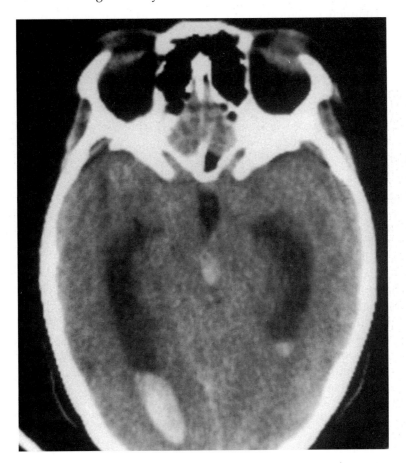

Figure A64

effacement of the sulci and compression of the lateral ventricles due to cerebral oedema. The diagnosis is that of subarachnoid haemorrhage and associated cerebral oedema.

All patients considered fit for surgery who have a non-traumatic subarachnoid haemorrhage require either conventional cerebral angiography or magnetic resonance angiography to locate the site of the aneurysm or arteriovenous malformation.

There is an increased incidence of communicating hydrocephalus in patients who suffer subarachnoid haemorrhage. This CT brain scan of another patient (Figure A64) who has had a subarachnoid haemorrhage demonstrates blood in the dilated third ventricle and the occipital horns. The dilated ventricles indicate that this patient has communicating hydrocephalus.

Answer 65

There is complete opacification of the right lung. The mediastinum is shifted to the right, as demonstrated by the position of the endotracheal tube and the course of the nasogastric tube. There is an increase in the reticulonodular shadows adjacent to the left hilum and the left lower zone. The appearances are those of complete right lung collapse, with changes of bronchiolitis in the left lung.

Lobar and lung collapse are well-recognized complications of bronchiolitis, due to mucus plugs obstructing the airways. During complete lung collapse, compensatory hyperinflation of the contralateral lung often herniates across the midline.

Answer 66

The long line lies superior to the clavicle and its tip is in front of or behind the trachea. There is blunting of the right costophrenic angle and effacement of the normal right hemidiaphragm/lung interface (i.e. silhouette sign) due to a large rightsided pleural effusion. The position of the long line is too high to be in the subclavian vein. The pleural effusion is a hydrothorax from fluid injected into the long line.

Appreciation of the normal venous anatomy on the chest radiograph is important (see Question and Answer 8) so that the route of long lines can be correctly interpreted. If in doubt, a linogram (Figure A66) is necessary which in this case demonstrates a false lumen around the long line. Venous access is via the transverse cervical vein (arrowed).

Answer 67

The distance between the posterior surface of the atlas and the anterior surface of the odontoid process is 10 mm in this case, the normal for an adult being no

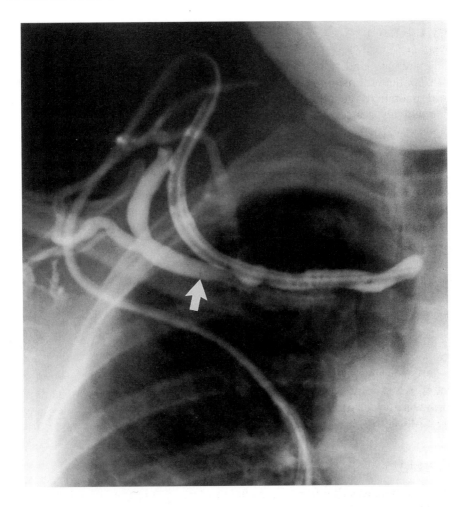

Figure A66

more than 3 mm. There is discontinuity of the spinolaminar line at the atlantoaxial level.

These appearances are consistent with rupture of the transverse ligament of the atlas, a complication of rheumatoid arthritis in this case. Other arthritides that cause atlantoaxial subluxation include psoriatic arthropathy, juvenile chronic arthritis, systemic lupus erythematosus and ankylosing spondylitis. It may occur as a complication of trauma or a retropharyngeal abscess. Congenital causes include trisomy 21, Morquio's syndrome and congenital hypoplasia and aplasia of the odontoid process.

Knowledge of atlantoaxial subluxation is important prior to anaesthesia so that neck flexion and the subsequent risk of neurological complications can be avoided.

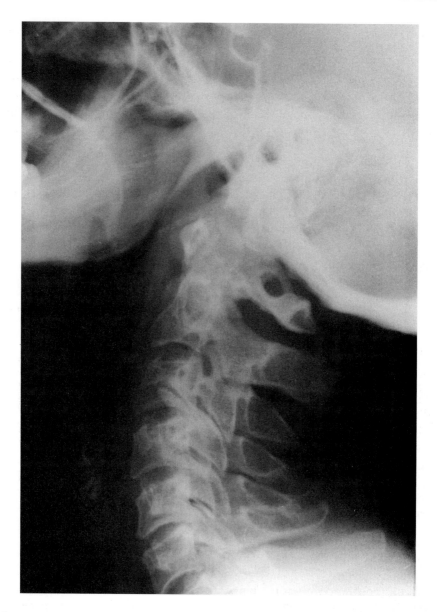

Figure A67

Answer 68

There is a curvilinear airfilled space in the lower left hemithorax, with absence of the normal diaphragmatic contour, and there is atelectasis of the left lower lobe. There is displacement of the heart to the right. These are the classic appearances of a ruptured left hemidiaphragm following blunt abdominal trauma. The large air bubble is the gastric fundus. Do not consider this to be a loculated pneumothorax requiring a chest drain!

The diagnosis of a ruptured hemidiaphragm relies upon the herniation of abdominal contents at the time of imaging. Rupture of the hemidiaphragm with visceral herniation can be masked or mimicked by superimposed pathology at the lung bases: eventration of the hemidiaphragm, post-traumatic phrenic nerve palsy, subphrenic fluid collection, acute gastric distension, loculated haemopneumothorax, chronic oesophageal hernias, post-traumatic lung cysts, atelectasis and pulmonary contusion. The next investigation of choice is a barium swallow and meal. In the case of gastric herniation, the stomach traverses the diaphragm and is situated within the left hemithorax, as demonstrated in another patient with a post-traumatic ruptured left hemidiaphragm (Figure A68).

Answer 69

The heart is enlarged and there is mediastinal widening. The trachea is deviated to the right. There are bilateral pleural effusions, the largest being on the

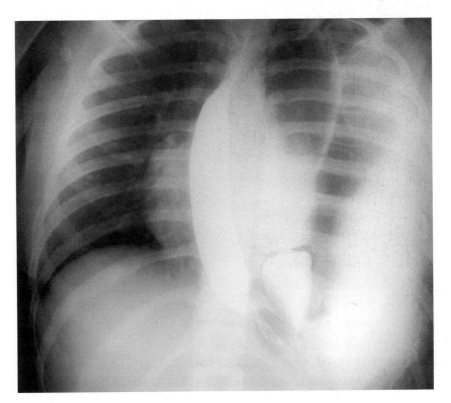

Figure A68

left. The large bulge along the right atrial border is due to a massively dilated ascending aorta.

The contrast-enhanced CT scan at the origin of the aortic root shows a 9 cm diameter ascending aortic aneurysm (arrows) and a compressed superior vena cava (open arrow). The descending aorta is of normal diameter. There is collapse of the left lower lobe and partial collapse of the right middle lobe which also enhances with contrast. An intimal flap is faintly demonstrated in the ascending aorta (curved arrow). There are large collections of pericardial and pleural fluid, likely to be due to leaking blood.

Thoracic aorta dissection is divided into two types: Type A in which the dissection occurs in the ascending aorta and Type B which begins at or distal to the ligamentum arteriosum and extends distally. Type A requires surgical treatment because of the risk of dissection into the pericardial space, as in this case. Type B can be treated medically.

Answer 70

The Swan-Ganz catheter takes a course to the left of the trachea and enters the right atrium via the coronary sinus. This indicates that a persistent left supe-

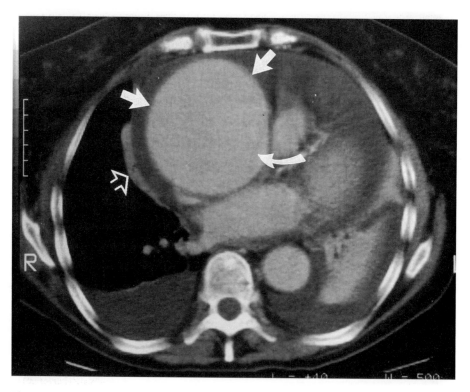

Figure A69

rior vena cava has been traversed. There is a widening of the superior mediastinum due to haemorrhage. Patchy consolidation is seen throughout both lungs consistent with the diagnosis of adult respiratory distress syndrome. The injection of a small quantity of non-ionic contrast medium under fluoroscopic control will demonstrate the location of the tip of the Swan–Ganz catheter if it is felt necessary to use the one traversing the persistent left superior vena cava.

The chest radiograph (Figure A70) taken prior to the one in Figure Q70 demonstrates two Swan-Ganz catheters, one in each of the superior vena cavae. A persistent left superior vena cava is an anatomical variant seen in 0.3% of the population. It can occur in isolation but there is usually a right superior vena cava. The left superior vena cava drains into the right atrium via the coronary sinus.

Answer 71

The pancreas is enlarged and has lost its normal surrounding fat. A large inflammatory mass or phlegmon is displacing the stomach anteriorly and extends down into the left anterior pararenal space. There are strands of in-

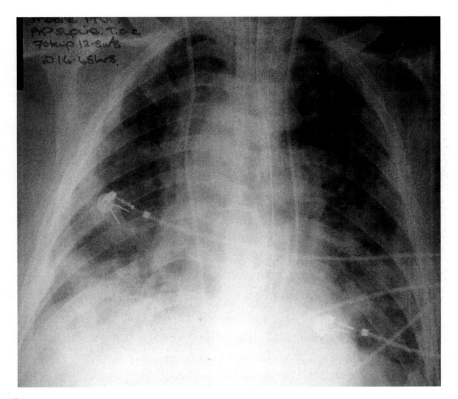

Figure A70

creased attenuation within the mesenteric fat, left perinephric fat and in the left loin subcutaneous fat due to inflammation. These are the computed tomographic appearances of severe pancreatitis. The serum amylase confirmed this. There are 11 prognostic indicators: age greater than 55 years, admission blood glucose greater than 11 mmol/l, admission white cell count greater than 16 x10^9/l, admission serum aspartate transaminase level exceeding 250 IU/l, admission serum lactic dehydrogenase level greater than 350 IU/l. The following six prognostic signs that have significance during the next 48 hours are a serum calcium level less than 2 mmol/l, arterial PO$_2$ less than 60 mmHg, an increase in blood urea greater than 1.8 mmol/l, a base deficit greater than 4 mEq/l, a decrease in haematocrit greater than 10% and fluid sequestration greater than 6l. Patients with less than three of these prognostic signs have a mortality rate of 1%, with three or four signs 15%, with five or six signs 40% and with seven or more signs, nearly 100%.

A CT scan at the level of the superior mesenteric artery shows a normal pancreas (arrows) (Figure A71). CT is able to demonstrate the morphological range of this disease from minimal inflammation to the tissue necrosis, haemorrhage and inflammatory cells of a phlegmon. Pancreatic pseudocysts and abscess are identifiable and can be aspirated and drained with CT guidance.

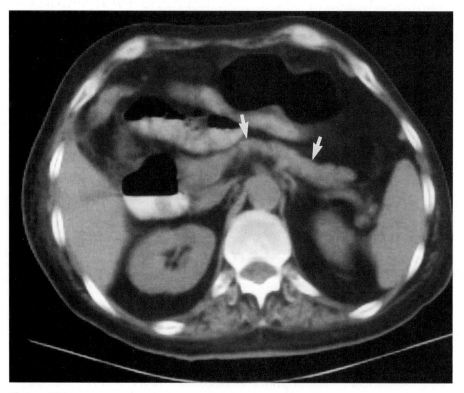

Figure A71

Answer 72

This 28 year old man was found at autopsy to have ruptured his aorta at the ligamentum arteriosum. The signs of aortic rupture on this radiograph include superior mediastinal widening with a leftsided paratracheal haematoma, loss of the normal aortic arch contour and deviation of the trachea to the right. Other radiological signs not present in this case may include nasogastric tube displacement to the right and depression of the left main bronchus. Associated findings include fracture of the upper ribs and an apical cap of blood over the apex of the left lung. With these chest radiographic signs and a haemodynamically stable patient an aortic angiogram is indicated which, if it proves positive, requires immediate thoracotomy and repair. There is bilateral patchy consolidation due to lung contusion.

Answer 73

There is opacification of the right hemithorax and 3 mm of fluid is demonstrated lateral to the right lung. This is the appearance of a supine pleural effusion which has occurred immediately post procedure, so this is a large haemothorax. The position of the long line is difficult to identify as the radiograph is slightly underpenetrated. As this is an immediate long line complication, laceration of the subclavian vein is likely and a repair of it should be considered if the blood loss continues. The position of the tip needs to be assessed with a more penetrated film, a lateral radiograph or a linogram.

A right lateral radiograph (Figure A73) shows that the long line (arrow) lies anterior to the superior vena cava. A large hydro/haemothorax is noted.

Answer 74

The tip of the endotracheal tube lies within the right lower lobe bronchus. There is collapse of the left lung and right upper lobe with crowding of the appropriate ribs and effacement of the mediastinal outline (silhouette sign). There is aeration of the right lower lobe. Management would include correct positioning of the tip of the endotracheal tube followed by suction and physiotherapy.

Answer 75

There are patchy regions of consolidation throughout both lungs, the largest having a diameter of approximately 6 cm. These are the appearances of pulmonary infarcts. In this case, the relative polycythaemia has contributed to the sickle cell crisis. The tip of the long line lies in the right internal jugular vein. These patients are at particular risk of *Streptococcus pneumoniae* infections because of autosplenectomy. Transtracheal aspirates should be sent for culture and antibiotics commenced if infection is suspected clinically.

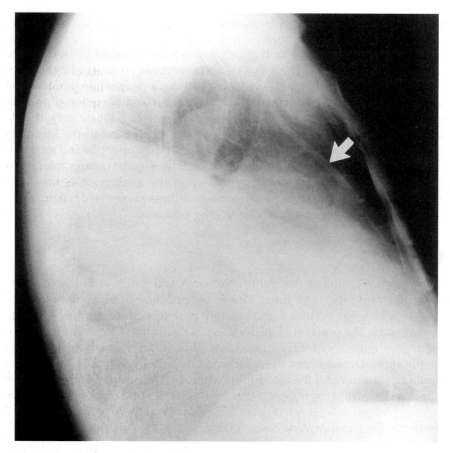

Figure A73

Answer 76

The barium remains in the pleural space, mainly in the region of the right cardiophrenic angle. Parts of the right sixth and seventh ribs have been surgically removed. There is a rightsided pleural effusion and partial collapse of the right lower lobe. This patient has an oesophagopleural fistula which is due to a breakdown of his gastro-oesophageal anastomosis. Water-soluble contrast medium, rather than barium, should be used for a contrast swallow when there is the possibility of an oesophageal leak. The extravasated barium may remain for a considerable period of time and may stimulate granuloma formation.

Answer 77

The patient is rotated. There is extensive surgical emphysema. The tip of the endotracheal tube is in a satisfactory position. However, there is mediastinal shift to the right. There are bilateral chest drains and the vessels of the right lung are just visible through the surgical emphysema. The lung vessels of the left lung are not identifiable. The appearances are those of a persistent left pneumothorax despite a well-positioned chest drain, indicating a traumatic bronchopleural fistula. The management includes a double lumen tube insertion and selective ventilation of the right lung, whilst air is aspirated from the left pneumothorax. Bronchoscopy showed a tear of the trachea and left main bronchus. The tracheal tear was repaired, but the extensive bronchial tear necessitated a left pneumonectomy.

An unresponsive pneumothorax following trauma, despite adequate drainage tube placement, suggests a major pulmonary, bronchial, tracheal, laryngeal or oesophageal laceration and necessitates prompt endoscopy of the airways and oesophagus.

Answer 78

There is localized bilateral consolidation in the regions of the superior segments of both lower lobes, with sparing of the apices and lower zones. A 5.5 cm thinwalled cyst is situated in the right lower lobe (Figure A78). The tip of

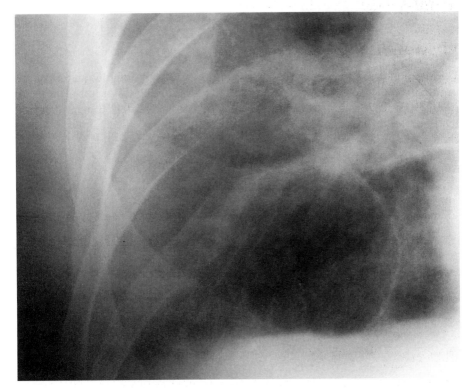

Figure A78

the Swan-Ganz catheter is too peripheral down a branch of the right pulmonary artery. The tip of the right central line is in the internal jugular vein. The right lower lobe cyst indicates interstitial emphysema due to barotrauma from mechanical ventilation. The ventilatory pressures should be reduced to the minimum needed. These cysts vary in size from day to day. They can herald a pneumothorax. The bilateral lower lobe superior segment consolidation is due to aspiration pneumonia from the postoperative site ooze bypassing a poorly sealing tracheostomy cuff and tracking into the first posteriorly positioned segmental bronchus orifice in a supine patient (the apical segments of the lower lobes).

Answer 79

There is air within the fascial planes of the chest wall and neck (surgical emphysema). The right visceral pleural outline lies approximately 2.5 cm medial to the lateral part of the ribs. The tip of the chest drain is seen lateral to the ribs. The mediastinum is shifted to the left. There is patchy consolidation throughout both lungs, consistent with adult respiratory distress syndrome. The chest drain has fallen out and urgently needs to be replaced and securely sutured in place.

Answer 80

There is a large rightsided tension pneumothorax, with the mediastinum being displaced to the left and the right hemidiaphragm inverted. There are nodular opacities and an air bronchogram within the left lung indicating hyaline membrane disease. The tension pneumothorax was caused by mechanical ventilation and requires immediate drainage.

Appendix

Indications for cardiac and thoracic radiology

Adapted from *Making the Best Use of a Department of Radiology*, 3rd ed, 1995, Royal College of Radiologists.

Clinical situation	Investigation	Guideline	Comment
Central chest pain ? myocardial infarction,	CXR	Indicated	CXR must not delay admission. CXR can assess heart size, pulmonary oedema, etc. and can exclude other causes
myocardial damage	NM	Specialized investigation	After stress ECG. Myocardial perfusion study detects and quantifies areas of ischaemia. NM can also assess LV function for prognostic purposes. US is also used here. MRI starting to be used and, because of high accuracy and no X-irradiation, this is likely to increase.
?Aortic dissection	CXR	Indicated	but mainly to exclude other causes; rarely diagnostic.
– acute	CT/US	Indicated	Seek advice from local radiologists. Much variation. Modern CT systems provide very accurate results. Often coupled with transthoracic US or, better, transoesophageal US. MRI probably the most accurate test and increasingly used, despite some logistic problems and constraints with some life-support systems. Angiography rarely necessary unless above examinations are equivocal.
Aortic dissection – chronic	MRI	Specialized investigation	MRI best investigation to assess change in longitudinal extent.

CXR – chest radiography; NM – nuclear medicine; CT – computed tomagraphy; US – ultrasound; MRI – magnetic resonance imaging

Clinical situation	Investigation	Guideline	Comment
?Pulmonary embolus	NM	Indicated	Interpreted along with contemporary CXR. Equivocal findings (e.g.intermediate probability) may necessitate pulmonary angiography or spiral CT for clarification. Some centres use US to show thrombus in leg veins for further proof.
Non-specific chest pain	CXR	Six week suggestion	Conditions such as Tietze's disease will not show on XR. Main purpose isreassurance.
Chest trauma (mild)	CXR	Not routinely indicated	Showing a rib fracture does not alter management. PA CXR only if pneumothorax suspected.
Pre-employment or screening medicals	CXR	Not indicated	Not justified except in a few high-risk categories (e.g .at-risk immigrants with no recent XR). Some have to be done for occupational (e.g. divers) or emigration purposes (UK category 2).
Preoperative	CXR	Not routinely	Exceptions before cardiopulmonary surgery, suspected malignancy or possible TB. Anaesthetists may also request CXRs for dyspnoeic patients and those with known cardiac disease. Many patients with cardiorespiratory disease have a recent CXR available; a repeat CXR may not be needed.
Heart disease/ hypertension follow-up	CXR	Not routinely indicated	Only if signs or symptoms have changed.
Upper respiratory tract infection	CXR	Not indicated	

Clinical situation	Investigation	Guideline	Comment
Chronic obstructive airways disease/asthma – follow-up	CXR	Not indicated	Only if signs or symptoms have changed.
Pneumonia – adults – follow-up	CXR	Indicated	To confirm clearing, etc. Pointless to re-examine at less than 7–10 day intervals as clearing can be slow (especially in the elderly). See also section on Children.
Pericarditis?	CXR	Indicated	but may be normal and cannot determine volume or effect of effusion.
Pericardial effusion?	US	Indicated	Extremely accurate; may be needed urgently for ?tamponade; can show best access for drainage. CT sometimes needed for ?calcification, etc.
Pleural effusion?	CXR	Indicated	but small effusions can be missed, especially on a frontal CXR
	US	Indicated	to prove fluid consistency; to guide aspiration. CT occasionally needed for better localization of solid components, etc.
Haemoptysis	CXR	Indicated	PA plus lateral view. Most centres proceed to bronchoscopy;
	CT	Specialized investigation	some use CT first.

Clinical situation	Investigation	Guideline	Comment
Children			
Acute chest infection	CXR	Not routinely indicated	Many infections in the community only involve the bronchi. If signs/symptoms suggest lung infection, a CXR should show/rule out parenchymal involvement or collapse. With simple consolidation follow-up is not required after good clinical response to treatment. If there is lobar collapse, segmental consolidation or poor response to treatment, follow-up is essential. Consider CXR as part of 'septic screen'; some children have pneumonia without clinical signs. Recurrent
cough/wheeze	CXR	Indicated	Children with recurrent chest infection +/− asthma usually have normal CXRs but may have bronchial wall thickening which implies chronicity.
?Inhaled foreign body	CXR	Indicated	Inspiratory plus expiratory CXRs required for evidence of air trapping. Decubitus views can help. Chest screening in young children (although high radiation dose). History of inhalation often not clear. Bronchoscopy if in doubt, even with normal CXR.
Sudden unexplained wheeze	CXR	Indicated	May be due to inhaled foreign body. Again, consider expiratory CXR.
Preoperative chest	CXR	Not indicated	As for adults.

References

Armstrong P, Wilson AG, Dee P. *Imaging of Diseases of the Chest,* 2nd edition. Mosby Year Book, St. Louis, 1994.

Barash PG, Cullen BF, Stoelting RK. *Clinical Anaesthesia.* Lippincott, London, 1989.

Collins VJ. *Principles of Anaesthesiology,* 3rd edition. Lea and Febiger, Philadelphia, 1993.

Fraser RG, Paré JAP, Paré PD, Fraser RS, Genereux GP. *Diagnosis of the Diseases of the Chest,* 3rd edition. WB Saunders, Philadelphia, 1988.

Goodman LR, Putman CE. *Intensive Care Radiology: Imaging of the Critically Illl,* 2nd edition. WB Saunders, Philadelphia, 1983.

Grainger RG, Allison DJ, Margulis AR, Steiner RE. *Diagnostic Radiology,* 2nd edition. Churchill Livingstone. Edinburgh, 1992.

Levy RC, Hawkins H, Barson WG. *Radiology in Emergency Medicine.* Mosby Year Book, St. Louis, 1986.

McCort JJ, Mindelzun RE. *Trauma Radiology.* Churchill Livingstone, New York, 1990.

Mirvis SE, Young JW. *Imaging in Trauma and Critical Care.* Williams and Wilkins, Baltimore, 1992.

Nunn JF, Utting JE, Brown BR. *General Anaesthesia,* 5th edition. Butterworth, London, 1989.

Sutton D. *Textbook of Radiology and Imaging,* 5th edition. Churchill Livingstone, Edinburgh, 1993.

Index